KETO MEAL PREP COOKB~
FOR BEGINNERS

KETOGENIC

HEAVEN

How To Cook Delicious Keto
Recipes While Counting Keto
Carbs and Practicing Clean Eating
For Vegetarians and Meat Lovers

PAULA HENRY

Table of Contents

PART I

Chapter 1: Meal Planning 101

Sticking to a diet is something that is not the easiest in the world. When it comes down to it, we struggle to change up our diets on a whim. It might be that for the first few days, you are able to stick to it and make sure that you are only eating those foods that are better for you, but over time, you will get to a point where you feel the pressure to cave in. You might realize that sticking to your diet is difficult and think that stopping for a burger on your way home won't be too bad. You might think that figuring out lunch or dinner is too much of a hassle, or you realize that the foods that you have bought forgot a key ingredient that you needed for dinner.

The good news is, you have an easy fix. When you are able to figure out what you are making for yourself for your meals well in advance, you stop having to worry so much about the foods that you eat, what you do with them, and what you are going to reach for when it's time to eat. You will be able to change up what you are doing so that you can be certain that the meals that you are enjoying are good for you, and you won't have to worry so much about the stress that goes into it. Let's take a look at what you need to do to get started with meal planning so that you can begin to do so without having to think too much about it.

Make a Menu

First, before you do anything, make sure that you make a menu! This should be something that you do on your own, or you should sit down with your family to ask them what they prefer. If you can do this, you will be able to ensure that you've got a clear-cut plan. When you have a menu a week in advance, you save yourself time and money because you know that all of your meals will use ingredients that are similar, and you won't have to spend forever thinking about what you should make at any point in time.

Plan around Ads

When you do your menu, make it a point to glance through the weekly ads as well. Typically, you will find that there are plenty of deals that you can make use of that will save you money.

Go Meatless Once Per Week

A great thing to do that is highly recommended on the Mediterranean Diet is to have a day each week where you go meatless for dinner. By doing so, you will realize that you can actually cut costs and enjoy the foods more at the same time. It is a great way to get that additional fruit and veggie content into your day, and there are plenty of healthy options that are out there for you. You just have to commit to doing so. In the meal plans that you'll see below, you will notice that there will be a meatless day on Day 2 every week.

Use Ingredients That You Already Have On Hand

Make it a point to use ingredients that you already have on hand whenever possible. Alternatively, make sure that all of the meals that you eat during the week use very similar ingredients. When you do this, you know that you're avoiding causing any waste or losing ingredients along the way, meaning that you can save money. The good news is, on the Mediterranean diet, there are plenty of delicious meals that enjoy very similar ingredients that you can eat.

Avoid Recipes that Call for a Special Ingredient

If you're trying to avoid waste, it is a good idea for you to avoid any ingredients in meals that are not going to carry over to other meals during your weekly plan. By avoiding doing so, you can usually save yourself that money for that one ingredient that would be wasted. Alternatively, if you find that you really want that dish, try seeing if you can freeze some of it for later. When you do that, you can usually ensure that your special ingredient at least didn't go to waste.

Use Seasonal Foods

Fruits and veggies are usually cheaper when you buy them in season, and even better, when you do so, you will be enjoying a basic factor of the Mediterranean diet just by virtue of enjoying the foods when they are fresh. Fresher foods are usually tastier, and they also tend to carry more vitamins and minerals because they have not had the chance to degrade over time.

Make Use of Leftovers and Extra Portions

One of the greatest things that you can do when it comes to meal planning is to make use of your leftovers and make-ahead meals. When you do this regularly, making larger portions than you need, you can then use the extras as lunches and dinners all week long, meaning that you won't have to be constantly worrying about the food that you eat for lunch. We will use some of these in the meal plans that you will see as well.

Eat What You Enjoy

Finally, the last thing to remember with your meal plan is that you ought to be enjoying the foods that are on it at all times. When you ensure that the foods that you have on your plate are those that you actually enjoy, sticking to your meal plan doesn't become such a chore, and that means that you will be able to do better as well with your own diet. Your meal plan should be loaded up with foods that you are actually excited about enjoying. Meal planning and dieting should not be a drag—you should love every moment of it!

Chapter 2: 1 Month Meal Plan

This meal plan is designed to be used for one month to help you simplify making sure that you have delicious meals to eat without having to think. These meals are fantastic options if you don't know where to start but want to enjoy your Mediterranean diet without much hassle. For each of the five weeks included, you will get one breakfast recipe, one lunch recipe, one dinner recipe, and one snack recipe to make meal planning a breeze. So, give these recipes a try! Many of them are so delicious, you'll want to enjoy them over and over again!

Week 1: Success is no accident—you have to reach for it

Mediterranean Breakfast Sandwich

Serves: 4

Time: 20 minutes

Ingredients:

- Baby spinach (2 c.)

- Eggs (4)

- Fresh rosemary (1 Tbsp.)

- Low-fat feta cheese (4 Tbsp.)

- Multigrain sandwich thins (4)

- Olive oil (4 tsp.)

- Salt and pepper according to preference

- Tomato (1, cut into 8 slices)

Instructions:

1. Preheat your oven. This recipe works best at 375° F. Cut the sandwich things in half and brush the insides with half of your olive oil. Place the things on a baking sheet and toast for about five minutes or until the edges are lightly browned and crispy.

2. In a large skillet, heat the rest of your olive oil and the rosemary. Use medium-high heat. Crack your eggs into the skillet one at a time. Cook until the whites have set while keeping the yolks runny. Break the yolks and flip the eggs until done.

3. Serve by placing spinach in between two sandwich thins, along with two tomato slices, an egg, and a tablespoon of feta cheese.

Greek Chicken Bowls

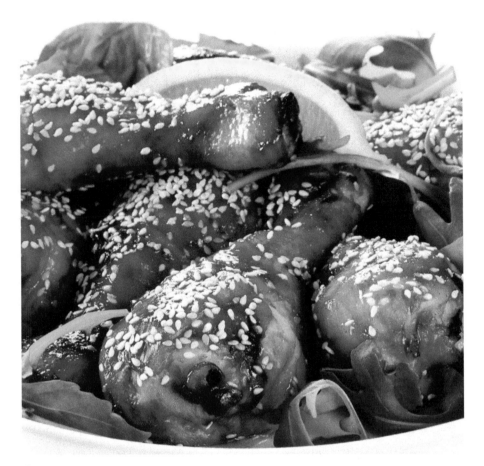

Serves: 4

Time: 20 minutes

Ingredients:

- Arugula (4 c.)
- Chicken breast tenders (1 lb.)

- Cucumber (1, diced)
- Curry powder (1 Tbsp.)
- Dried basil (1 tsp.)
- Garlic powder (1 tsp.)
- Kalamata olives (2 Tbsp.)
- Olive oil (1 Tbsp.)
- Pistachios (0.25 c., chopped)
- Red onion (half, sliced)
- Sunflower seeds (0.25 c.)
- Tzatziki sauce (1 c.)

Instructions:

1. In a bowl, mix in the chicken tenders, curry powder, dried basil, and garlic powder. Make sure to coat the chicken evenly.
2. Heat one tablespoon of olive oil over medium-high. Add the chicken and cook for about four minutes on each side. Remove from the pan and set aside to cool.
3. Place one cup of arugula into four bowls. Toss in the diced cucumber, onion, and kalamata olives.
4. Chop the chicken and distribute evenly between the four bowls.
5. Top with tzatziki sauce, pistachio seeds, and sunflower seeds.

Ratatouille

Serves: 8

Time: 1 hour 30 minutes

Ingredients:

- Crushed tomatoes (1 28 oz. can)
- Eggplants (2)
- Fresh basil (4 Tbsp., chopped)
- Fresh parsley (2 Tbsp., chopped)
- Fresh thyme (2 tsp.)
- Garlic cloves (4, minced and 1 tsp, minced)
- Olive oil (6 Tbsp.)
- Onion (1, diced)
- Red bell pepper (1, diced)
- Roma tomatoes (6)
- Salt and pepper to personal preference
- Yellow bell pepper (1, diced)
- Yellow squashes (2)
- Zucchinis (2)

Instructions:

1. Get your oven ready. This recipe works best at 375° F.
2. Slice the tomatoes, eggplant, squash, and zucchini into thin rounds and set them to the side.

3. Heat up two tablespoons of olive oil in an oven safe pan using medium-high heat. Sauté your onions, four cloves of garlic, and bell peppers for about ten minutes or when soft. Add in your pepper and salt along with the full can of crushed tomatoes. Add in two tablespoons of basil. Stir thoroughly.

4. Take the vegetable slices from earlier and arrange them on top of the sauce in a pattern of your choosing. For example, a slice of eggplant, followed by a slice of tomato, squash, and zucchini, then repeating. Start from the outside and work inward to the center of your pan. Sprinkle salt and pepper overtop the veggies.

5. In a bowl, toss in the remaining basil and garlic, thyme, parsley, salt, pepper, and the rest of the olive oil. Mix it all together, and spoon over the veggies.

6. Cover your pan and bake for 40 minutes. Uncover and then continue baking for another 20 minutes.

Snack Platter

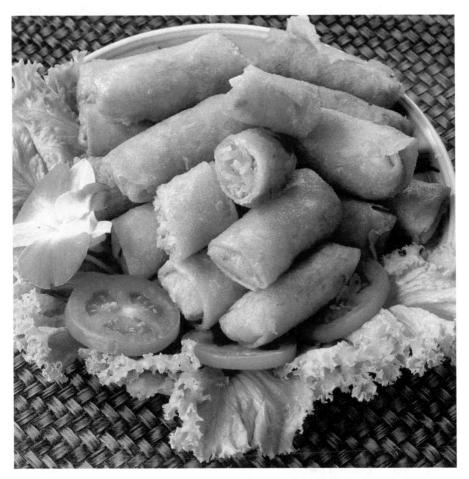

Serves: 6

Time:

Ingredients:

Rosemary Almonds

- Butter (1 Tbsp.)

- Dried rosemary (2 tsp.)
- Salt (pinch)
- Whole almonds (2 c.)

Hummus

- Chickpeas (1 15 oz. can, drained and rinsed)
- Garlic clove (1, peeled)
- Lemon (half, juiced)
- Olive oil (2 Tbsp.)
- Salt and pepper according to personal preference
- Tahini (2 Tbsp.)
- Water (2 Tbsp.)

Other sides

- Bell pepper (1, sliced)
- Cucumber (1, sliced)
- Feta cheese (4 oz, cubed)
- Kalamata olives (handful, drained)
- Pepperoncini peppers (6, drained)
- Pitas (6, sliced into wedges)
- Small fresh mozzarella balls (18)
- Soppressata (6 oz.)
- Sweet cherry peppers (18)

Instructions:

1. To get started, make your rosemary almonds. Take a large skillet and place it on a burner set to medium heat. Start melting the butter in, then toss in the almonds, rosemary and a bit of salt. Toss the nuts on occasion to ensure even coating.

2. Cook the almonds for roughly ten minutes, getting them nicely toasted. Set the almonds off to the side to let them cool.

3. Now you'll set out to make the hummus. Take a blender or food processor and toss in the hummus ingredients. Blend until you get a nice, smooth paste. If you find that your paste is too thick, try blending in a bit of water until you get the desired consistency. Once you have the right consistency, taste for seasoning and adjust as necessary.

4. Pour and scrape the hummus into a bowl and drizzle in a bit of olive oil. Set it off to the side to get the rest of the platter going.

5. Grab the sweet cherry peppers and stuff them with the little balls of mozzarella. Arrange a platter in any pattern you like. If serving for a party or family, try keeping each snack in its own little segment to keep things looking neat.

Week 2: Self-belief and effort will take you to what you want to achieve

Breakfast Quesadilla

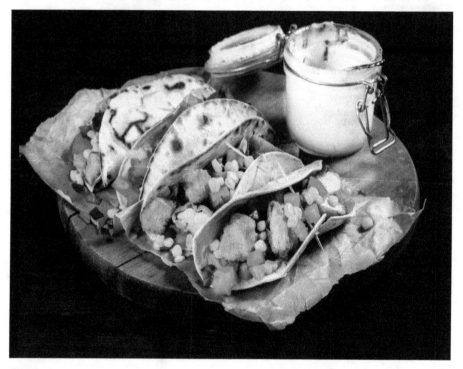

Serves: 1

Time: 10 minutes

Ingredients:

- Basil (handful)
- Eggs (2)
- Flour tortilla (1)

- Green pesto (1 tsp.)
- Mozzarella (0.25 c.)
- Salt and pepper according to personal preference
- Tomato (half, sliced)

Instructions:

1. Scramble your eggs until just a little runny. Remember, you will be cooking them further inside the quesadilla. Season with salt and pepper.
2. Take the eggs and spread over half of the tortilla.
3. Add basil, pesto, mozzarella cheese, and the slices of tomato.
4. Fold your tortilla and toast on an oiled pan. Toast until both sides are golden brown.

Greek Orzo Salad

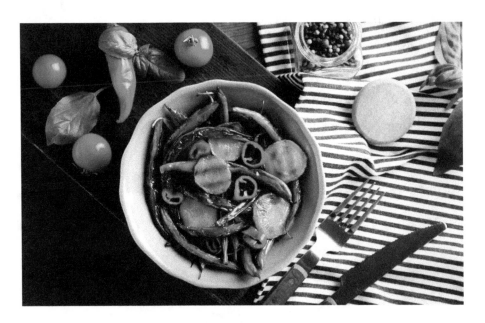

Serves: 6

Time: 25 minutes

Ingredients:

- Canned chickpeas (1 c., drained and rinsed)
- Dijon mustard (0.5 tsp)
- Dill (0.33 c., chopped)
- Dried oregano (1 tsp)
- English cucumber (half, diced)
- Feta cheese crumbles (0.5 c.)
- Kalamata olives (0.33 c., halved)
- Lemon (half, juice and zest)
- Mint (0.33 c., chopped)
- Olive oil (3 Tbsp.)
- Orzo pasta (1.25 c. when dry)
- Roasted red pepper (half, diced)
- Salt and pepper to taste
- Shallot (0.25 c., minced)
- White wine vinegar (2 Tbsp.)

Instructions:

1. Prepare the orzo according to the packaging details. Once the orzo is al dente, drain it and rinse until it drops to room temperature.
2. In a bowl, toss all the ingredients together until thoroughly incorporated.

One Pot Mediterranean Chicken

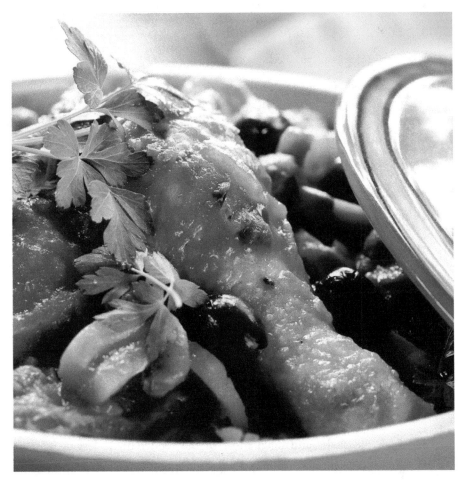

Serves: 4

Time: 1 hour

Ingredients:

- Chicken broth (3 c.)
- Chicken thighs (3, bone in, skin on)

- Chickpeas (1 15 oz can, drained and rinsed)
- Dried oregano (0.5 tsp.)
- Fresh parsley (2 Tbsp., chopped)
- Garlic cloves (2, minced)
- Kalamata olives (0.75 c., halved)
- Olive oil (2 tsp.)
- Onion (1, finely diced)
- Orzo pasta (8 ounces uncooked)
- Roasted peppers (0.5 c., chopped)
- Salt and pepper according to personal preference

Instructions:

1. Prepare your oven at 375°. Heat your olive oil in a large skillet over medium-high heat.
2. Season the chicken with salt and pepper on both sides. Toss the chicken into the skillet and cook for five minutes on each side, or until golden in color. Remove the chicken.
3. Take the skillet and drain most of the rendered fat, leaving about a teaspoon. Add the onion and cook for five minutes. Toss in the garlic and cook for an additional minute.
4. Now you will want to add the orzo, roasted peppers, oregano, chickpeas, and olives into the pan. Add in salt and pepper.
5. Place the thighs on top of the orzo and pour in the chicken broth.
6. Bring to a boil, then cover and place in the oven. Bake for 35 minutes or until chicken has cooked through. Top with parsley and serve.

Mediterranean Nachos

Serves: 6

Time: 10 minutes

Ingredients:

- Canned artichoke hearts (1 c., rinsed, drained, and dried)
- Canned garbanzo beans (0.75 c., rinsed, drained, and dried)
- Feta cheese (0.5 c., crumbled)
- Fresh cilantro (2 Tbsp., chopped)
- Pine nuts (2.5 Tbsp.)
- Roasted red peppers (0.5 c., dried)
- Sabra Hummus (half of their 10 oz. container)
- Tomatoes (0.5 c., chopped)
- Tortilla chips (roughly half a bag)

Instructions:

1. Get your oven ready by setting it to 375°F. In a baking pan, layer the tortilla chips, and spread hummus over them evenly. Top with garbanzo beans, red peppers, artichoke hearts, feta cheese, and pine nuts.
2. Bake for about five minutes or until warmed through. Remove the baking pan and top the nachos with fresh cilantro and tomatoes. Serve and enjoy.

Week 3: The harder you work, the greater the success

Breakfast Tostadas

Serves: 4

Time: 15 minutes

Ingredients:

- Beaten eggs (8)
- Cucumber (0.5 c., seeded and chopped)
- Feta (0.25 c., crumbled)
- Garlic powder (0.5 tsp)
- Green onions (0.5 c., chopped)
- Oregano (0.5 tsp)
- Red Pepper (0.5 c., diced)
- Roasted red pepper hummus (0.5 c.)
- Skim milk (0.5 c.)
- Tomatoes (0.5 c., diced)
- Tostadas (4)

Instructions:

1. In a large skillet, cook the red pepper for two minutes on medium heat until softened. Toss in the eggs, garlic powder, milk, oregano, and green onions. Stir constantly until the egg whites have set.
2. Top the tostadas with hummus, egg mixture, cucumber, feta, and tomatoes.

Roasted Vegetable Bowl

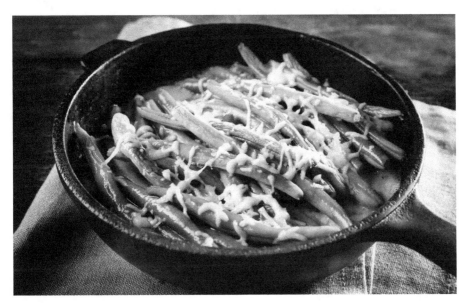

Serves: 2

Time: 45 minutes

Ingredients:

- Crushed red pepper flakes (a pinch)
- Fresh parsley (1 Tbsp., chopped)
- Kalamata olives (0.25 c.)
- Kale (1 c., ribboned)
- Lemon juice (1 Tbsp.)
- Marinated artichoke hearts (0.25 c., drained and chopped)
- Nutritional yeast (1 Tbsp.)
- Olive oil (1 Tbsp., then enough to drizzle)
- Salt and pepper to taste

- Spaghetti squash (half, seeds removed)
- Sun-dried tomatoes (2 Tbsp., chopped)
- Walnuts (0.25 c., chopped)

Instructions:

1. Get your oven ready by setting it to 400° F. Take a baking sheet and blanket it with parchment paper.
2. Take the squash half and place it on the parchment paper. Drizzle olive oil over the side that is cut, and season with salt and pepper. Turn it over so it is facing cut side down and bake for 40 minutes. It is ready when it is soft.
3. Remove the squash shell, and season with a bit more salt and pepper.
4. Stack the kale, artichoke hearts, walnuts, sun-dried tomatoes, and kalamata olives on the squash.
5. Squeeze the lemon juice over and drizzle olive oil. Finish with chopped parsley and a bit of crushed red pepper flakes.

Mediterranean Chicken

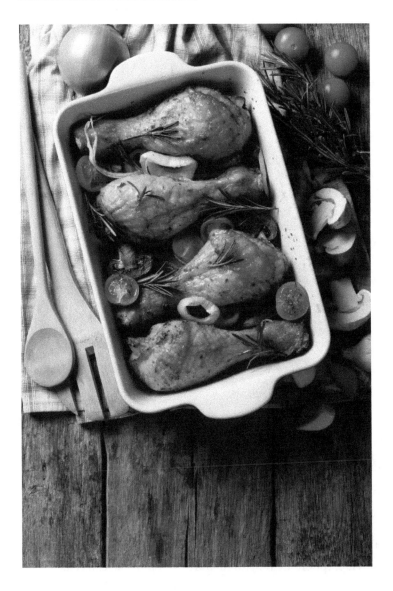

Serves: 4

Time: 40 minutes

Ingredients:

- Chicken breasts (1 lb., boneless, skinless)
- Chives (2 Tbsp., chopped)
- Feta cheese (0.25 c., crumbled)
- Garlic (1 tsp., minced)
- Italian seasoning (1 tsp.)
- Lemon juice (2 Tbsp.)
- Olive oil (2 Tbsp., and 1 Tbsp.)
- Salt and pepper according to personal preference
- Tomatoes (1 c., diced)

Instructions:

1. Pour in two tablespoons of olive oil, the lemon juice, salt, pepper, garlic, and Italian seasoning in a resealable plastic bag. Add in the chicken, seal and shake to coat the chicken.
2. Allow the chicken to marinate for at least 30 minutes in the refrigerator.
3. Heat the rest of the olive oil in a pan over medium heat.
4. Place the chicken on the pan and cook for five minutes on each side, or until cooked through.
5. In a bowl, mix the tomatoes, chives, and feta cheese. Season with salt and pepper.
6. When serving, spoon the tomato mixture on top of the chicken.

Baked Phyllo Chips

Serves: 2

Time: 10 minutes

Ingredients:

- Grated cheese (your choice)
- Olive oil (enough to brush with)
- Phyllo sheets (4)
- Salt and pepper according to personal preference

Instructions:

1. Get your oven ready by setting it to 350° F. Brush olive oil over a phyllo sheet generously. Sprinkle grated cheese and your seasoning on top.
2. Grab a second sheet of your phyllo and place it on top of the first one. Again, brush with olive oil and sprinkle cheese and seasoning on top.
3. Repeat this process with the remaining sheets of phyllo. Top the stack with cheese and seasoning.
4. Once complete, cut the stack of phyllo into bite-sized rectangles. A pizza cutter may be helpful here.
5. Grab a baking sheet and blanket it with some parchment paper. Take your phyllo rectangles and place them on the parchment paper.
6. Bake in the oven for about seven minutes or until they reach a golden color.
7. Remove them from the oven and allow them to cool before serving.

Week 4: You don't need perfection—you need effort

Mini Omelets

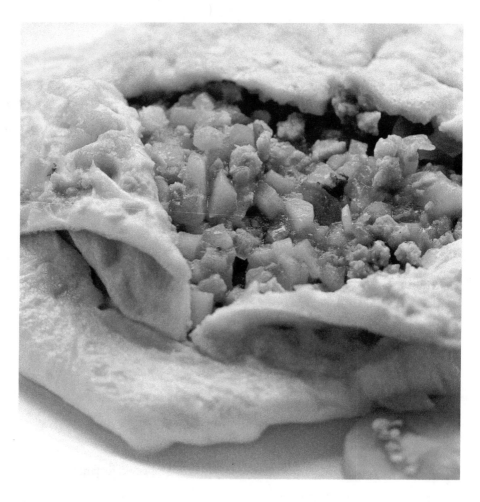

Serves: 8

Time: 40 minutes

Ingredients:

- Cheddar cheese (0.25 c., shredded)
- Eggs (8)
- Half and half (0.5 c.)
- Olive oil (2 tsps.)
- Salt and pepper according to personal preference
- Spinach (1 c., chopped)

Instructions:

1. Get your oven ready by setting it to 350° F. Prepare a muffin pan or ramekins by greasing them with olive oil.
2. In a bowl, beat the eggs and dairy until you have a fluffy consistency.
3. Stir in the cheese and your seasonings. Pour in the spinach and continue beating the eggs.
4. Pour the egg mixture into your ramekins or muffin pan.
5. Bake the omelets until they have set, which should be roughly 25 minutes. Remove them from the oven and allow them to cool before serving.

Basil Shrimp Salad

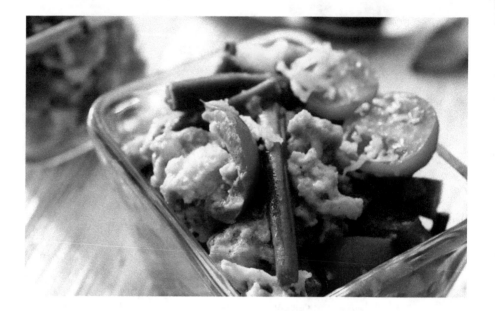

Serves: 2

Time: 40 minutes

Ingredients:

- Dried basil (1 tsp.)
- Lemon juice (1 Tbsp.)
- Olive oil (1 tsp.)
- Romaine lettuce (2 c.)
- Shrimp (12 medium or 8 large)
- White wine vinegar (0.25 c.)

Instructions:

1. Whisk together the white wine vinegar, olive oil, lemon juice, and basil. Stick your shrimp in the marinade for half an hour.
2. Take the marinade and shrimp and cook in a skillet over medium heat until cooked through.
3. Allow the shrimp to cool along with the juice and pour into a bowl. Toss in the romaine lettuce and mix well to get the flavor thoroughly infused in the salad. Serve.

Mediterranean Flounder

Serves: 4

Time: 40 minutes

Ingredients:

- Capers (0.25 c.)
- Diced tomatoes (1 can)
- Flounder fillets (1 lb.)
- Fresh basil (12 leaves, chopped)
- Fresh parmesan cheese (3 Tbsp., grated)
- Garlic cloves (2, chopped)
- Italian seasoning (a pinch)
- Kalamata olives (0.5 c., pitted and chopped)
- Lemon juice (1 tsp.)

- Red onion (half, chopped)
- White wine (0.25 c.)

Instructions:

1. Set your oven to 425° F. Take a skillet and pour in enough olive oil to sauté the onion until soft. Cook on medium-high heat.
2. Toss in the garlic, Italian seasoning, and tomatoes. Cook for an additional five minutes.
3. Pour in the wine, capers, olives, lemon juice, and only half of the basil you chopped.
4. Reduce the heat to low and stir in the parmesan cheese. Simmer for ten minutes or until the sauce has thickened.
5. Place the flounder fillets in a baking pan and pour the sauce over top. Sprinkle the remaining basil on top and bake for 12 minutes.

Nutty Energy Bites

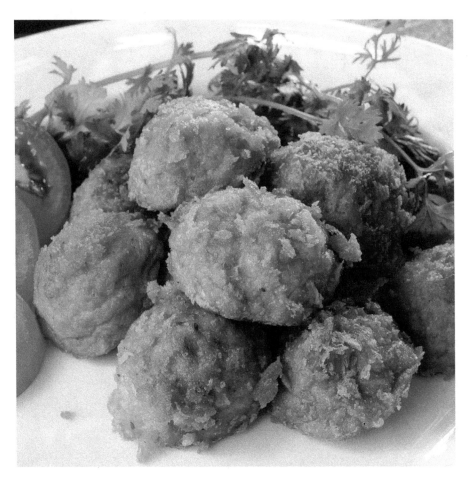

Serves: 10

Time: 10 minutes

Ingredients:

- Dried dates (1 c., pitted)
- Almonds (0.5 c.)

- Pine nuts (0.25 c.)
- Flaxseeds (1 Tbsp., milled) Porridge oats (2 Tbsp.)
- Pistachios (0.25 c., coarsely ground)

Instructions:

1. Take the dates, pine nuts, milled flaxseeds, almonds, and porridge oats and pour them into a food processor or blender. Mix until thoroughly incorporated.
2. Using a tablespoon, scoop the mixture and roll it between your hands until you have a small, bite-sized ball. Do this until you have used the entirety of the dough. This recipe should be enough for about ten.
3. On a plate, sprinkle your ground pistachios. Take the energy balls and roll them on the pistachio grounds, making sure to coat them evenly. Serve or store in the refrigerator.

Week 5: Transformation Happens One Day at a Time

Mediterranean Breakfast Bowl

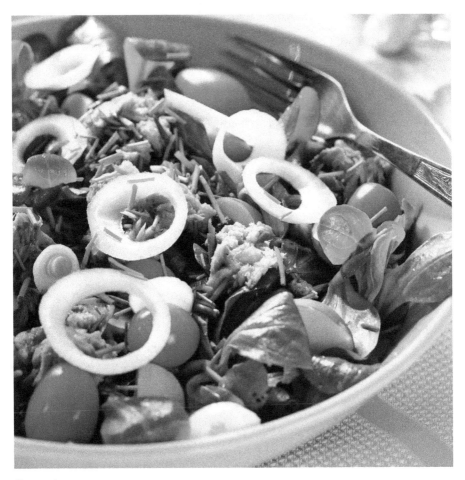

Serves: 1

Time: 25 minutes

Ingredients:

- Artichoke hearts (0.25 c., chopped)
- Baby arugula (2 c.)
- Capers (1 Tbsp.)
- Egg (1)
- Feta (2 Tbsp., crumbled)
- Garlic (0.25 tsp)
- Kalamata olives (5, chopped)
- Lemon thyme (1 Tbsp., chopped)
- Olive oil (0.5 Tbsp.)
- Pepper (0.25 tsp)
- Sun-dried tomatoes (2 Tbsp., chopped)
- Sweet potato (1 c., cubed)

Instructions:

1. Take your olive oil and, when hot, pan fry your sweet potatoes for 5-10 minutes until they have softened. Then, sprinkle on the seasonings.
2. Place arugula into a bowl, then top with potatoes, then everything but the egg.
3. Prepare the egg to your liking and serve.

Chicken Shawarma Pita Pockets

Serves: 6

Time: 40 minutes

Ingredients:

- Cayenne (0.5 tsp)
- Chicken thighs (8, boneless, skinless, bite-sized pieces)
- Cloves (0.5 tsp, ground)
- Garlic powder (0.75 Tbsp.)
- Ground cumin (0.75 Tbsp.)
- Lemon juice (1 lemon)
- Olive oil (0.33 c.)
- Onion (1, sliced thinly)
- Paprika (0.75 Tbsp.)
- Salt
- Turmeric powder (0.75 Tbsp.)

To serve:

- Pita pockets (6)
- Tzatziki sauce
- Arugula
- Diced tomatoes
- Diced onions
- Sliced Kalamata olives

Instructions:

1. Combine all spices. Then, place all chicken, already diced, into the bowl. Coat well, then toss in onions, lemon juice, and oil. Mix well and let marinade for at least 3 hours, or overnight.

2. Preheat the oven to 425 F. Allow chicken to sit at room temperature a few minutes. Then, spread it on an oiled sheet pan. Roast for 30 minutes.

3. To serve, fill up a pita pocket with tzatziki, chicken, arugula, and any toppings you prefer. Enjoy.

Turkey Mediterranean Casserole

Serves: 6

Time: 35 minutes

Ingredients:

- Fusilli pasta (0.5 lbs.)
- Turkey (1.5 c., chopped)
- Sun dried tomatoes (2 Tbsp., drained)
- Canned artichokes (7 oz., drained)
- Kalamata olives (3.5 oz., drained and chopped)
- Parsley (0.5 Tbsp., chopped and fresh)
- Basil (1 T, fresh)
- Salt and pepper to taste
- Marinara sauce (1 c.)

- Black chopped olives (2 oz., drained)
- Mozzarella cheese (1.5 c., shredded)

Instructions:

1. Warm your oven to 350 F. Prepare your pasta according to the directions, drain, and place into a bowl. Prepare your basil, parsley, olives, tomatoes, artichokes, and other ingredients.

2. Mix together the pasta with the turkey, tomatoes, olives, artichokes, herbs, seasoning, and marinara sauce. Give it a good mix to incorporate all of the ingredients evenly.

3. Take a 9x13 oven-safe dish and layer in the first half of your pasta mixture. Then, sprinkle on half of your mozzarella cheese. Top with the rest of the pasta, then sprinkle on the chopped black olives as well. Spread the rest of the shredded cheese on top, then bake it for 20-25 minutes. It is done when the cheese is all bubbly and the casserole is hot.

Heirloom Tomato and Cucumber Toast

Serves: 2

Time: 5 minutes

Ingredients:

- Heirloom tomato (1, diced)
- Persian cucumber (1, diced)
- Extra virgin olive oil (1 tsp)
- Oregano (a pinch, dried)
- Kosher salt and pepper
- Whipped cream cheese (2 tsp)
- Whole grain bread (2 pieces)
- Balsamic glaze (1 tsp)

Instructions:

4. Combine the tomato, cucumber, oil, and all seasonings together.
5. Spread cheese across bread, then top with mixture, followed by balsamic glaze.

Chapter 3: Maintaining Your Diet

Sticking to a diet can be tough. You could see that other people are having some great food and wish that you could enjoy it too. You might realize that you miss the foods that you used to eat and feel like it's a drag to not be able to enjoy them. When you are able to enjoy the foods that you are eating, sticking to your diet is far easier. However, that doesn't mean that you won't miss those old foods sometimes. Thankfully, the Mediterranean diet is not a very restrictive one—you are able to enjoy foods in moderation that would otherwise not be allowed, and because of that, you can take the slice of cake at the work party, or you can choose to pick up a coffee for yourself every now and then. When you do this, you're not doing anything wrong, so long as you enjoy food in moderation.

Within this chapter, we are going to take a look at several tips that you can use that will help you with maintaining your diet so that you will be able to stick to it, even when you feel like things are getting difficult. Think of this as your guide to avoiding giving in entirely—this will help you to do the best thing for yourself so that you can know that you are healthy. Now, let's get started.

Find Your Motivation

First, if you want to keep yourself on your diet, one of the best things that you can do is make sure that you find and stick to your motivation. Make sure that you know what it is in life that is motivating you. Are you losing weight because a doctor told you to? Fair enough—but how do you make that personal and about yourself? Maybe instead of looking at it as a purely health-related choice, look at it as something that you are doing because of yourself. Maybe you are eating better so that you are able to watch your children graduate or so that you can run after them at the park and stay healthy, even when it is hard to do so.

Remind Yourself Why You are Eating Healthily

When you find that you are struggling to eat healthily, remind yourself of why you are doing it in the first place. When you do this enough, you will begin to resist the urges easier than ever. Make it a point to tell yourself not to eat something a certain way. Take the time to remind yourself that you don't need to order that greasy pizza—you are eating better foods because you want to be there for your children or grandchildren.

Reminding yourself of your motivation is a great way to overcome those cravings that you may have at any point in time. The cravings that you have are usually strong and compelling, but if you learn to overcome them, you realize that they weren't actually as powerful as you thought they were. Defeat the cravings. Learn to tell yourself that they are not actually able to control you. Tell yourself that you can do better with yourself.

Eat Slowly

Now, on the Mediterranean diet, you should already be eating your meals with other people anyway. You should be taking the time to enjoy those meals while talking to other people and ensuring that you get that connection with them, and in doing so, you realize that you are able to do better. You realize that you are able to keep yourself under control longer, and that is a great way to defend and protect yourself from overeating.

When you eat slowly, you can get the same effect. Eating slowly means that you will have longer for your brain to realize that you should be eating less. When you are able to trigger that sensation of satiety because you were eating slowly, you end up eating fewer calories by default, and that matters immensely.

Keep Yourself Accountable

Don't forget that, ultimately, your diet is something that you must control on your own. Keep yourself accountable by making sure that you show other people what you are doing. If you are trying to lose weight, let them know, and tell them how you plan to do so. When you do this, you are able to remind yourself that other people know what you are doing and why—this is a great way to foster that sense of accountability because you will feel like you have to actually follow through, or you will be embarrassed by having to admit fault. You could also make accountability to yourself as well. When you do this, you are able to remind yourself that your diet is your own. Using apps to track your food and caloric intake is just one way that you can do this.

Remember Your Moderation

While it can be difficult to face a diet where you feel like you can't actually enjoy the foods that you would like to eat, the truth is that on the Mediterranean diet, you are totally okay to eat those foods that you like or miss if you do so in moderation. There is nothing that is absolutely forbidden on the Mediterranean diet—there are just foods that you should be restricting regularly. However, that doesn't mean that you can't have a treat every now and then.

Remembering to live in moderation will help you from feeling like you have to cheat or give up as well. When you are able to enjoy your diet and still enjoy the times where you want to enjoy your treats, you realize that there is actually a happy medium between sticking to the diet and deciding to quit entirely.

Identify the Difference between Hunger and Craving

Another great way to help yourself stick to your diet is to recognize that there is a very real difference between actually being hungry and just craving something to eat. In general, cravings are felt in the mouth—when you feel like you are salivating or like you need to eat something, but it is entirely in your head and mouth, you know that you have a craving. When you are truly hungry, you feel an emptiness in your stomach—you are able to know because your abdomen is where the motivation is coming from.

Being able to tell when you have a craving and when you are genuinely hungry, you can usually avoid eating extra calories that you didn't actually need. This is major—if you don't want to overeat, you need to know when your body actually needs something and when it just wants something. And if you find that you just want something, that's okay too—just find a way to move on from it. If you want to indulge a bit here and there, there's no harm in that!

Stick to the Meal Plan

When it comes to sticking to a diet, one of the easiest and most straightforward ways to do so is to just stick to your meal plan that you set up. You have it there for a reason—it is there for you to fall back on, and the sooner that you are willing to accept that, recognizing that ultimately, you can stay on track when you don't have to think about things too much, the better you will do. You will be able to succeed on your diet because you will know that you have those tools in place to protect you—they will be lined up to ensure that your diet is able to provide you with everything that you need and they will also be there so that you can know that you are on the right track.

Drink Plenty of Water

Another key to keeping yourself on track with your diet is to make sure that you drink plenty of water throughout the day. Oftentimes, we mistake our thirst with hunger and eat instead. Of course, if you're thirsty, food isn't going to really fix your problem, and you will end up continuing to mix up the sensation as you try to move past it. The more you eat, the thirstier you will get until you realize that you're full but still feeling "hungry." By drinking plenty of water any time that you think that you might want to eat, you will be able to keep yourself hydrated, and in addition, you will prevent yourself from unintentionally eating too much.

Eat Several Times Per Day

One of the best ways to keep yourself on track with your diet is to make sure that you are regularly eating. By eating throughout the day, making sure that you keep yourself full, it is easier to keep yourself strong enough to resist giving in to cravings or anything else. When you do this regularly, you will discover that you can actually keep away much of your cravings so that you are more successful in managing your diet.

Eating several times per day often involves small meals and snacks if you prefer to do so. Some people don't like doing this, but if you find that you're one of those people who will do well on a diet when you are never actually hungry enough to get desperate enough to break it, you will probably be just fine.

Fill Up on Protein

Another great way to protect yourself from giving in and caving on your diet is to make sure that you fill up on protein. Whether it comes from an animal or plant source, make sure that every time you eat, you have some sort of tangible protein source. This is the best way to keep yourself on track because protein keeps you fuller for longer. When you eat something that's loaded up with protein, you don't feel the need to eat as much later on. The protein is usually very dense, and that means that you get to resist feeling hungry for longer than you thought that you would.

Some easy proteins come from nuts—but make sure that you are mindful that you do not end up overeating during this process—you might unintentionally end up eating too many without realizing it. While you should be eating proteins regularly, make sure that you are mindful of calorie content as well!

Keep Only Healthy Foods

A common mistake that people make while dieting is that they end up caving when they realize that their home is filled up with foods that they shouldn't be eating. Perhaps you are the only person in your home that is attempting to diet. In this case, you may end up running into a situation where you have all sorts of non-compliant foods on hand. You might have chips for your kids or snacks that your partner likes to eat on hand. You may feel like it is difficult for you to stay firm when you have that to consider, and that means that you end up stuck in temptation.

One of the best ways to prevent this is to either cut all of the unhealthy junk out of your home entirely or make sure that you keep the off-limits foods in specific places so that you don't have to look at it and see it tempting you every time that you go to get a snack for yourself. By trying to keep yourself limited to just healthy foods, you will be healthier, and you will make better decisions.

Eat Breakfast Daily

Finally, make sure that breakfast is non-negotiable. Make sure that you enjoy it every single day, even if you're busy. This is where those make-ahead meals can come in handy; by knowing that you have to keep to a meal plan and knowing that you already have the food on hand, you can keep yourself fed. Breakfast sets you up for success or failure—if you want to truly succeed on your diet, you must make sure that you are willing to eat those healthier foods as much as possible, and you must get started on the right foot. Enjoy those foods first thing every day. Eat so that you are not ravenous when you finally do decide that it is time to sit down and find something to eat. Even if you just have a smoothie or something quick to eat as you go, having breakfast will help you to persevere.

PART II

Keto Recipes

The keto diet is a high-fat and low-carb diet that comes with various health benefits. It has been found that this diet can help you lose weight and improve the condition of your health. It might also show some positive effects on cancer, diabetes, Alzheimer's, and epilepsy. This diet's main aim is to reduce the intake of carbs drastically and replace the same with healthy fats. When you reduce the consumption of carbs, the body will enter a metabolic state known as ketosis. During ketosis, the body will try its best to burn the body fat for generating energy. It will also be turning the liver fat into ketones that supply energy to the brain.

A keto diet is a very effective way of losing weight. The best aspect of this diet is that you can lose bodyweight without counting calories. The reason behind this is that the diet will be so filling that you will not have frequent cravings. It has been found that people who follow a keto diet can lose 2.5 times more weight when compared to those people who follow a calorie-restrictive diet. The keto diet can also deal with type 2 diabetes, metabolic, and prediabetes syndrome. Some other benefits of the keto diet are:

- **Cancer:** This diet can help suppress the growth of tumors and might also help in treating various types of cancer.

- **Heart diseases:** The keto diet can help deal with various chronic heart conditions such as heart attack, stroke, and others.

- **Polycystic ovary:** This diet is well known for reducing insulin levels that can help in dealing with polycystic ovary.

There are certain food items that you will need to include while following this diet.

- **Fatty fish:** Trout, salmon, mackerel, tuna

- **Meat:** Steak, sausage, red meat, ham, chicken, bacon, turkey

- **Seeds and nuts:** Walnuts, almonds, pumpkin seeds, flax seeds, chia seeds

- **Oils:** Coconut oil, olive oil, avocado oil

A keto diet is an excellent option for all those who have diabetes, overweight or want to improve the health of their metabolism. I have included some tasty and easy keto recipes that you can include in your diet plan.

Chapter 1: Gourmet Recipes

If you are looking for some tasty keto gourmet recipes, this section has got what you are searching for. So, let's have a look at them.

Creamy Garlic Chicken

Total Prep & Cooking Time: Twenty-five minutes

Yields: Six servings

Nutrition Facts: Calories: 348 | Protein: 28g | Carbs: 6.3g | Fat: 22.3g | Fiber: 0.9g

Ingredients

- Two pounds of chicken breasts (sliced thinly)
- Two tbsps. of olive oil
- One cup of each
  - Heavy cream
  - Spinach (chopped)
- Half cup of each
  - Chicken stock
  - Parmesan cheese
  - Sun-dried tomatoes
- One tsp. of each
  - Italian seasoning
  - Garlic powder

Method:

1. Take an iron skillet and add olive oil in it. After the oil gets hot, add the chicken and cook for five minutes. Remove the pieces of chicken from the skillet. Keep aside.

2. Add chicken stock, heavy cream, Italian seasoning, garlic powder, and parmesan cheese in the skillet. Whisk the mixture on medium flame until the sauce thickens. Add tomatoes and spinach. Simmer the mixture for two minutes until the spinach wilts.

3. Addcooked chicken into the prepared sauce. Cook for two minutes.

4. Serve hot.

Mediterranean Lemon Herb Chicken Salad

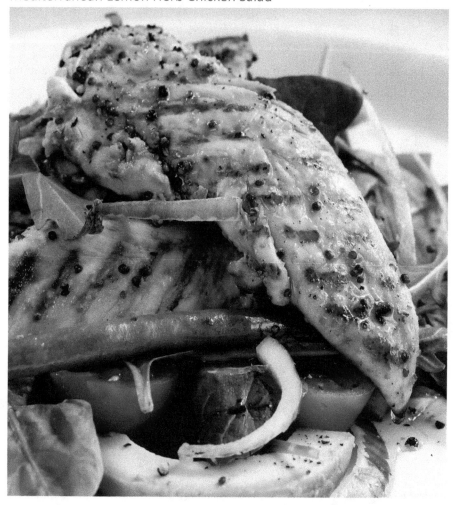

Total Prep & Cooking Time: Twenty-five minutes

Yields: Four servings

Nutrition Facts: Calories: 326 | Protein: 22.3g | Carbs: 12g | Fat: 20.1g | Fiber: 6.2g

Ingredients

- Two tbsps. of each
  - Olive oil
  - Water
  - Parsley (chopped)
  - Red wine vinegar
  - Basil (dried)
  - Garlic (minced)
- One lemon (juiced)
- One tsp. of each
  - Salt
  - Oregano
- One pound of chicken thighs

For the salad:

- Four cups of lettuce leaves (washed)
- One cucumber (diced)
- Two tomatoes (diced)
- One onion (sliced)
- One avocado (sliced)
- One-third cup of kalamata olives (sliced)
- Wedges of lemon (for serving)

Method:

1. Whisk all the marinade ingredients in a bowl. Pour half of the marinade in a shallow dish. Store the remaining marinade for the dressing.

2. Add the pieces of chicken in the marinade dish and marinate for half an hour.

3. Mix all the ingredients for the salad in a mixing bowl and keep aside.

4. Heat some oil in a grill pan. Add the marinated chicken and cook for five minutes on each side until browned on all sides.

5. Slice the chicken pieces.

6. Serve the salad with chicken from the top. Drizzle some of the marinade and serve with lemon wedges.

Garlic Butter Scallops and Steak

Total Prep & Cooking Time: Thirty minutes

Yields: Two servings

Nutrition Facts: Calories: 280 | Protein: 23.1g | Carbs: 1.2g | Fat: 1.3g | Fiber: 0.3g

Ingredients

- Two fillets of beef tenderloin
- Black pepper and kosher salt (according to taste)
- Three tbsps. of butter
- Ten sea scallops

For the sauce:

- Three garlic cloves (minced)
- Six tbsps. of butter (cubed)
- Two tbsps. of each
  - Chives (chopped)
  - Parsley (chopped)
- One tbsp. of lemon juice
- Two tsps. of lemon zest

- Black pepper and kosher salt (according to taste)

Method:

1. Take an iron skillet and heat it over medium flame for ten minutes.

2. Season the steak with pepper and salt.

3. Add two tbsps. of butter in the skillet. Add the steak and cook for six minutes on each side. Cook until the steak reaches your desired doneness.

4. Keep the steak aside and heat one tbsp. of butter in the skillet.

5. Remove the muscles from the small side of the scallops and wash them with cold running water.

6. Season the scallops with pepper and salt. Cook the scallops on each side for three minutes.

7. For making the sauce, add garlic and butter in a skillet. Stir for one minute. Add chives, lemon zest, parsley, and lemon juice. Add pepper and salt for seasoning.

8. Serve the scallops and steak with butter sauce from the top.

Fried Chicken

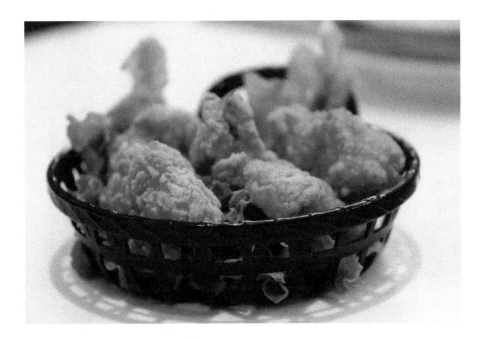

Total Prep & Cooking Time: Fifty minutes

Yields: Twelve servings

Nutrition Facts: Calories: 305 | Protein: 38.2g | Carbs: 0.6g | Fat: 12.3g | Fiber: 0.5g

Ingredients

- Four ounces of pork rinds
- Two tsps. of thyme (dried)

- One tsp. of each
    - Black pepper
    - Salt
    - Oregano (dried)
- Half tsp. of garlic powder
- One-third tsp. of paprika (smoked)
- Twelve chicken legs
- One large egg
- Two ounces of mayonnaise
- Three tbsps. of Dijon mustard

Method:

1. Crush the pork rinds for making powder texture. Leave some of the big pieces.

2. Preheat the oven at 200 degrees Celsius.

3. Mix salt, pork rinds, thyme, pepper, garlic powder, oregano, and paprika. Spread out the prepared mixture on a large flat dish.

4. Combine Dijon mustard, egg, and mayonnaise in a bowl. Dip the chicken legs in the egg mixture and then roll in the mixture of pork rind. Coat well.

5. Place the legs of chicken on a baking tray. Bake for forty minutes.

6. Serve hot.

Lime Chile Steak Fajitas

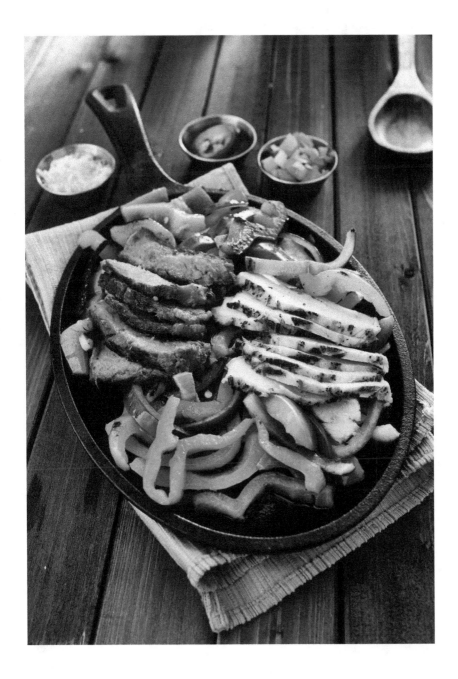

Total Prep & Cooking Time: Twenty-five minutes

Yields: Four servings

Nutrition Facts: Calories: 419 | Protein: 23.1g | Carbs: 12g | Fat: 25.6g | Fiber: 5.1g

Ingredients

For the marinade:

- Two tbsps. of olive oil
- One-third cup of lime juice
- Three tbsps. of cilantro (chopped)
- Two garlic cloves (chopped)
- One tsp. of brown sugar
- Three-fourth tsp. of chili flakes
- Half tsp. of cumin (ground)
- One tsp. of salt
- One pound of steak

For the fajitas:

- Three capsicums (different colors, sliced)
- One avocado (sliced)
- One onion (sliced)

For serving:

- Tortillas
- Sour cream

Method:

1. Combine all the marinade ingredients in a bowl. Keep aside half of the marinade. Pour the remaining marinade in a flat dish and marinate the steak.

2. Heat one tsp. of oil in a skillet. Add the steak and grill for five minutes on each side. Allow the steak to cool down for five minutes.

3. Wipe the skillet and brush some oil. Fry the capsicums along with the strips of onion. Add the reserved marinade, pepper, and salt.

4. For serving the steak, slice the steak. Arrange steak, sour cream, avocado, and cooked veggies in the tortillas. Serve with marinade and cilantro from the top.

Spaghetti Squash With Stuffed Lasagna

Total Prep & Cooking Time: Two hours

Yields: Four servings

Nutrition Facts: Calories: 280 | Protein: 23.1g | Carbs: 6.7g | Fat: 21.3g | Fiber: 0.2g

Ingredients

- One pound of Italian sausage
- One spaghetti squash
- One cup of pasta sauce (low-carb)
- One-fourth cup of ricotta
- One-third cup of mozzarella
- Half cup of parmesan
- Pepper and salt (according to taste)
- Parsley (for garnishing)

Method:

1. Cut spaghetti squash in half. Remove the seeds. Bake the squash in the oven with the cut side down in one inch of water. Bake for fifty minutes at 200 degrees Celsius.

2. Take a skillet and add the sausage. Cook until browned and add pasta sauce. Simmer for ten minutes and add seasonings.

3. Take out the baked squash and scrape the inside portion with the help of a fork. Add the squash strands in a bowl.

4. Combine the strands with ricotta, meat sauce, and cheese.

5. Stuff the squash shells with the mixture and arrange in a baking sheet. Top with mozzarella.

6. Bake the squash for fifteen minutes until the cheese melts.

7. Serve with parsley from the top.

Zucchini Boats With Stuffed Tuna

Total Prep & Cooking Time: Thirty minutes

Yields: Two servings

Nutrition Facts: Calories: 412 | Protein: 37.2g | Carbs: 23.2g | Fat: 18.3g | Fiber: 10.6g

Ingredients

- Two tsps. of avocado oil
- Half red bell pepper (diced)
- Two cans of wild tuna
- Half cup of salsa
- Two zucchinis
- Pepper and salt
- Half tsp. of cumin

For salsa:

- One avocado (cubed)
- One-fourth cup of cilantro (chopped)
- Three tbsps. of onion (minced)
- Two tsps. of lime juice

Method:

1. Take a frying pan and heat oil in it. Add diced pepper and sauté for two minutes. Remove the pepper and add tuna. Cook for four minutes.

2. Add salsa to the pan. Combine well.

3. Trim the zucchini ends. Slice them in half, lengthwise. Use a spoon for scraping out the flesh. Sprinkle some cumin, pepper, and salt.

4. Fill the zucchini shells with tuna mixture.

5. Preheat your oven at 200 degrees Celsius.

6. Bake the zucchini for twenty minutes.

7. Mix the ingredients for the salsa in a large small mixing bowl.

8. Serve the zucchini boats with salsa by the side.

Spinach and Goat Cheese Stuffed Breast of Chicken

Total Prep & Cooking Time: Forty-five minutes

Yields: Four servings

Nutrition Facts: Calories: 229 | Protein: 27.8g | Carbs: 4.9g | Fat: 13.7g | Fiber: 2.8g

Ingredients

- Four breasts of chicken
- Two tbsps. of olive oil
- Four cups of spinach
- Half tsp. of garlic powder
- Two ounces of goat cheese
- One onion (sliced)
- Eight ounces of bella mushrooms
- One tsp. of thyme
- Pepper and salt (for seasoning)

Method:

1. Heat the oven at 175 degrees Celsius.

2. Use a sharp knife for cutting slits on the upper side of the chicken breasts. Drizzle the breasts with olive oil, pepper, and salt. Keep aside.

3. Take a large skillet and heat half tbsp. of oil in it. Add spinach and cook for two minutes. Add garlic powder and cook until the spinach wilts.

4. Transfer spinach to a bowl. Add the goat cheese. Combine well.

5. Stuff the slits of the chicken breasts with the cheese and spinach mixture.

6. Heat one tbsp. of oil in the same skillet. Add mushrooms, onion, and thyme. Season with pepper and salt. Cook until the onions caramelize. Move the cooked veggies to a side to make some room for the chicken breasts.

7. Add the stuffed chicken breasts to the skillet.

8. Put the skillet in the oven. Bake for thirty minutes.

9. Serve hot.

Chapter 2: Quick and Easy Recipes

When you are short of time, opting for quick and easy recipes is the best option. So, I have included some easy recipes in this section that you can make without any hassle.

Antipasto Salad

Total Prep & Cooking Time: Thirty minutes

Yields: Two servings

Nutrition Facts: Calories: 510 | Protein: 36.8g | Carbs: 12.4g | Fat: 61g | Fiber: 10.6g

Ingredients

- Ten ounces of lettuce (chopped in pieces)
- Two tbsps. of parsley (chopped)
- Five ounces of mozzarella cheese (sliced)
- Three ounces of each
  - Salami (sliced thinly)
  - Prosciutto (sliced thinly)
- Four ounces of canned artichokes (quartered)
- Two cups of roasted red pepper
- One ounce of each
  - Sun-dried tomatoes (chopped)
  - Olives (sliced)
- One-third cup of basil

- One chili pepper (chopped)
- Half tbsp. of salt
- Four tbsps. of olive oil

Method:

1. Distribute the leaves of lettuce on serving plates or on a large dish.

2. Add parsley from the top.

3. Layer all the ingredients of antipasto.

4. In a bowl, mix chopped chili, basil, and salt. Crush the ingredients using a wooden spoon.

5. Sprinkle the crushed mixture over the salad and serve with olive oil from the top.

Feta Cheese and Chicken Plate

Total Prep & Cooking Time: Ten minutes

Yields: Two servings

Nutrition Facts: Calories: 810 | Protein: 63.3g | Carbs: 8.7g | Fat: 71g | Fiber: 3.2g

Ingredients

- Five-hundred grams of rotisserie chicken
- Two cups of feta cheese
- Two tomatoes
- Three cups of lettuce
- Ten olives
- One-third cup of olive oil
- Pepper and salt (according to taste)

Method:

1. Arrange chicken, lettuce, cheese, and olives on a plate. Slice the tomatoes and arrange them on the plate.

2. Sprinkle pepper and salt for seasoning.

3. Serve with olive oil from the top.

Note: If you do not want to use rotisserie chicken, you can cook the chicken from scratch.

Cheese Omelet

Total Prep & Cooking Time: Fifteen minutes

Yields: Two servings

Nutrition Facts: Calories: 797 | Protein: 37.2g | Carbs: 3.9g | Fat: 74.2g | Fiber: 0.1g

Ingredients

- Half cup of butter
- Six large eggs
- One cup of cheddar cheese (shredded)
- Pepper and salt (according to taste)

Method:

1. Break the eggs in a bowl. Add the cheese and whisk. Season with pepper and salt.

2. Take a medium-sized pan and melt some butter in it. Add the whisked egg mixture and allow it to set for two minutes.

3. Reduce the flame and cook for four minutes on each side. Add the leftover cheese.

4. Fold the omelet in half. Cook for one more minute.

5. Serve hot.

Baked Salmon and Pesto

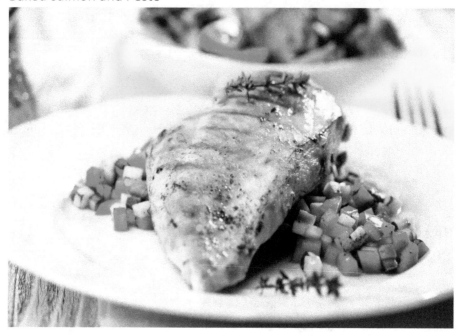

Total Prep & Cooking Time: Thirty minutes

Yields: Four servings

Nutrition Facts: Calories: 625 | Protein: 48.3g | Carbs: 3.2g | Fat: 89g | Fiber: 0.7g

Ingredients

- Four tbsps. of pesto
- One cup of mayonnaise
- Half cup of Greek yogurt
- Pepper and salt (according to taste)

For the salmon:

- Four fillets of salmon
- Four tbsps. of green pesto
- Pepper and salt (for seasoning)

Method:

1. Grease a baking dish with some oil. Place the fillets of salmon on the dish with the skin-side down. Spread green pesto on the fillets and season with pepper and salt.

2. Bake the salmon for thirty minutes at 200 degrees Celsius.

3. Stir the ingredients for the sauce in a bowl.

4. Serve the salmon with sauce from the top.

Pork Chops and Blue Cheese Sauce

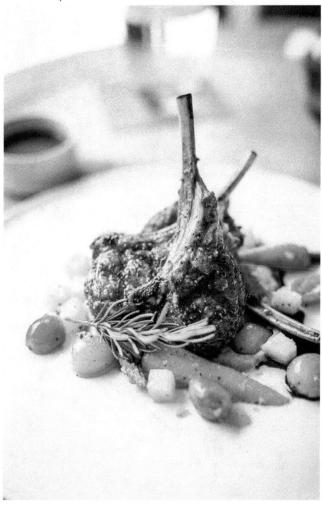

Total Prep & Cooking Time: Twenty minutes

Yields: Four servings

Nutrition Facts: Calories: 669 | Protein: 53.2g | Carbs: 4.3g | Fat: 60.1g | Fiber: 1.6g

Ingredients

- Two cups of blue cheese
- One cup of whipping cream (heavy)
- Four pork chops
- Seven ounces of green beans
- Two tbsps. of butter
- Pepper and salt

Method:

1. Crumble the blue cheese in a pot. Place the pot over medium flame and allow the cheese to melt.

2. Add whipping cream in the melted cheese and mix well. Simmer for two minutes.

3. Season the chops using pepper and salt.

4. Take an iron skillet and heat some oil in it. Add the chops and cook for four minutes on each side.

5. Add the juices from the pan in the sauce and stir.

6. Trim the beans. Heat some oil butter in the skillet and sauté the beans for two minutes.

7. Serve the pork chops with cheese sauce from the top and beans by the side.

Green Pepper and Pork Stir-Fry

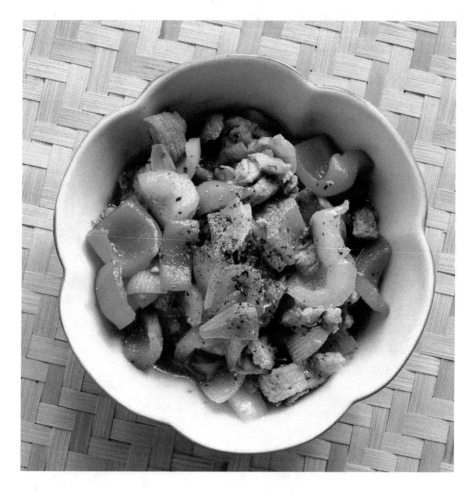

Total Prep & Cooking Time: Twenty-five minutes

Yields: Two servings

Nutrition Facts: Calories: 678 | Protein: 31.2g | Carbs: 5.3g | Fat: 71.3g | Fiber: 4.6g

Ingredients

- Four ounces of butter
- Four-hundred grams of pork shoulder (cut in strips)
- Two bell pepper (green, sliced)
- Two scallions (sliced)
- Half cup of almond
- One tsp. of chili paste
- Pepper and salt

Method:

1. Heat butter in a wok. Add the meat strips in the butter and cook for five minutes until browned.

2. Add the chili paste along with veggies. Cook for two minutes. Add pepper and salt.

3. Serve the stir-fry with almonds from the top.

Broccoli With Fried Chicken

Total Prep & Cooking Time: Thirty minutes

Yields: Two servings

Nutrition Facts: Calories: 633 | Protein: 30.1g | Carbs: 5.3g | Fat: 64.3g | Fiber: 3.6g

Ingredients

- Nine ounces of broccoli
- One cup of butter
- Ten ounces of chicken thighs (boneless)
- Pepper and salt
- Half cup of mayonnaise

Method:

1. Rinse the broccoli thoroughly under running water. Trim the florets along with the stem.

2. Heat some butter in a pan.

3. Season the chicken thighs. Add the chicken to the pan and cook them for five minutes on all sides.

4. Add some more butter in the pan and add the broccoli. Toss the broccoli and chicken and cook for two minutes.

5. Serve with mayonnaise from the top.

Fried Eggs With Pork and Kale
Total Prep & Cooking Time: Twenty-five minutes

Yields: Three servings

Nutrition Facts: Calories: 910 | Protein: 24g | Carbs: 7.6g | Fat: 89g | Fiber: 6.3g

Ingredients

- One cup of kale
- Three ounces of butter
- Six ounces of bacon or pork belly (smoked)
- One ounce of walnuts
- Four large eggs
- Pepper and salt

Method:

1. Chop the kale and wash them under cold water.

2. Melt some butter in a skillet and cook the kale for two minutes until the edges are slightly browned.

3. Remove kale from the skillet and keep aside. Add bacon or pork belly in the same skillet and sear until crispy.

4. Add the kale in the skillet along with walnuts. Toss the ingredients.

5. Heat butter in another pan and fry the eggs sunny side up. Add pepper and salt for seasoning.

6. Serve the eggs with kale mixture by the side.

Chapter 3: Sweet Recipes

Even when you are on a diet, you don't have to compromise on satisfying your sweet tooth. So, I have included some easy to make sweet keto recipes in this section.

Sugar Cinnamon Donuts

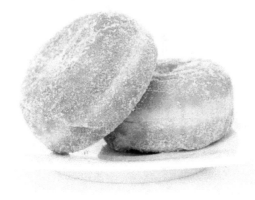

Total Prep & Cooking Time: Twenty-five minutes

Yields: Twelve servings

Nutrition Facts: Calories: 82 | Protein: 2.3g | Carbs: 1.9g | Fat: 7.8g | Fiber: 0.3g

Ingredients

- Two eggs
- One-fourth cup of almond milk
- One-fourth tsp. of apple cider vinegar

- One tsp. of vanilla extract
- Two tbsps. of butter
- One-third cup of sweetener
- One cup of fine almond flour
- Half tbsp. of coconut flour
- One tsp. of cinnamon (ground)
- One and a half tsp. of baking powder
- Half tsp. of baking soda
- Half cup of salt

For sugar cinnamon coating:

- One-fourth cup of granulated erythritol
- One tsp. of cinnamon (ground)
- Two tbsps. of butter

Method:

1. Whisk together almond milk, eggs, butter, vinegar, vanilla extract, and sweetener. Combine until smooth.

2. Combine coconut flour, almond flour, baking powder, cinnamon, salt, and baking soda in a bowl. Add all the dry ingredients slowly to the mixture of wet ingredients. Stir well until combined.

3. Transfer the donut batter into a donut pan.

4. Bake the donuts for fifteen minutes at 175 degrees Celsius.

5. Take out the donuts and keep aside for cooling.

6. Stir together cinnamon and sweetener in a bowl.

7. Melt the butter in a pan.

8. Take the donuts and dunk them in the butter. Roll the donuts in the cinnamon coating.

Mug Brownie

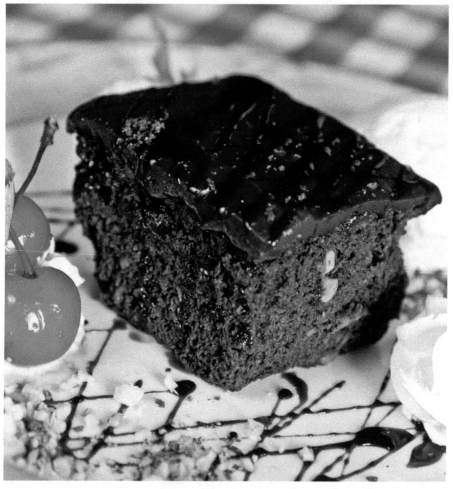

Total Prep & Cooking Time: Ten minutes

Yields: Two servings

Nutrition Facts: Calories: 194 | Protein: 7.9g | Carbs: 7.6g | Fat: 16.5g | Fiber: 6.7g

Ingredients

- Two tbsps. of almond flour
- One tbsp. of each
  - Granulated sweetener
  - Cocoa powder
  - Almond butter
  - Chocolate chips
- One-eighth tsp. of baking powder
- Three tbsps. of milk

Method:

1. Use a cooking spray for greasing cereal bowls or mugs.

2. Combine the listed dry ingredients. Mix properly.

3. Mix milk and almond butter in a separate bowl and mix well.

4. Combine the dry and wet ingredients. Mix well. Add the chocolate chips and fold well.

5. Pour the batter in the cereal bowls. Bake for six minutes.

6. Enjoy your brownie from the bowl.

Mini Cheesecake

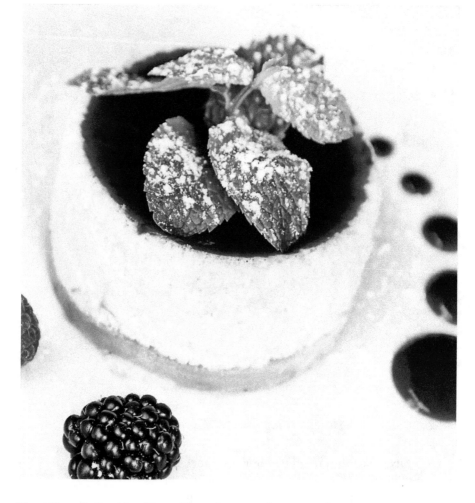

Total Prep & Cooking Time: Three hours and twenty minutes

Yields: Six servings

Nutrition Facts: Calories: 230 | Protein: 4.7g | Carbs: 5.1g | Fat: 19.6g | Fiber: 1.8g

Ingredients

For the crust:

- Half cup of almond flour
- Two tbsps. of sweetener
- Half tsp. of cinnamon
- Two tbsps. of butter (melted)

For the filling:

- Six ounces of cream cheese (softened)
- Five tbsps. of sweetener
- One-fourth cup of sour cream
- Half tsp. of vanilla extract
- One egg
- Two tsps. of cinnamon (ground)

For the frosting:

- One tbsp. of butter (softened)
- Three tbsps. of confectioners sweetener
- One-fourth tsp. of vanilla extract
- Two tsps. of heavy cream

Method:

1. Heat the oven at 175 degrees Celsius. Line a small muffin pan with six silicone liners.

2. Whisk almond flour, cinnamon, and sweetener in a bowl. Add melted butter and mix well.

3. Divide the prepared crust among the muffin cups. Press the crust to the bottom. Bake in the oven for five minutes.

4. Beat three tbsps. of sweetener along with the cream cheese in a bowl. Add vanilla, egg, and sour cream. Beat well.

5. Reduce oven temperature to 160 degrees Celsius.

6. Whisk cinnamon and butter in a bowl.

7. Add three-fourth tbsp. of cheese mixture into the muffin cups. Sprinkle cinnamon mixture from the top.

8. Bake the muffins for fifteen minutes. Refrigerate the muffins for two hours.

9. Beat powdered sweetener and butter in a bowl. Add heavy cream and vanilla extract. Mix well.

10. Transfer the frosting to a zip-lock bag and cut a small hole at the corner.

11. Add frosting over the cheesecakes.

Keto Fudge

Total Prep & Cooking Time: One hour

Yields: Twelve servings

Nutrition Facts: Calories: 158 | Protein: 0.1g | Carbs: 0.6g | Fat: 17.9g | Fiber: 0.7g

Ingredients

- One cup of coconut oil
- One-fourth cup of each
  - Cocoa powder
  - Erythritol (powdered)
- One tsp. of vanilla extract
- One-eighth tsp. of sea salt
- Sea salt

Method:

1. Use parchment paper for lining a glass baking dish.

2. Beat sweetener and coconut oil using a hand blender. Make sure the mixture is fluffy.

3. Add vanilla extract, cocoa powder, and salt. Combine well.

4. Pour the fudge mixture in the lined dish. Smoothen the top using a spoon or spatula.

5. Refrigerate the fudge for forty minutes until it solidifies.

6. Use a sharp knife to run along the edges of the dish for taking out the fudge.

7. Cut in small cubes and serve.

Peanut Butter Hearts

Total Prep & Cooking Time: Thirty minutes

Yields: Twenty servings

Nutrition Facts: Calories: 91 | Protein: 5.1g | Carbs: 7.1g | Fat: 6.7g | Fiber: 5.2g

Ingredients

- Two cups of peanut butter
- Three-fourth cup of any sticky sweetener
- One cup of coconut flour
- One and a half cup of chocolate chips

Method:

1. Use parchment paper for lining a large glass tray.

2. Combine sticky sweetener with peanut butter on the stovetop. Combine the mixture until it melts completely.

3. Add the coconut flour and combine. In case the batter is very thin, you can add more flour.

4. Make twenty balls from the dough. Use a heart-shaped cookie cutter for pressing the dough balls for making heart shape.

5. Arrange the hearts on the lined glass tray and refrigerate.

6. Melt the chocolate chips and dip the hearts in the melted chocolate.

7. Refrigerate again for twenty minutes until firm.

Peanut Butter and White Chocolate Blondies

Total Prep & Cooking Time: Three hours and thirty-five minutes

Yields: Sixteen servings

Nutrition Facts: Calories: 102 | Protein: 3.2g | Carbs: 2.2g | Fat: 9.3g | Fiber: 1.9g

Ingredients

- Half cup of each
    - Peanut butter
    - Sweetener of your choice
- Four tbsps. of butter (softened)
- Two large eggs
- One tsp. of vanilla extract
- Three tbsps. of cocoa butter (melted)
- One-fourth cup of almond flour
- One tbsp. of coconut flour
- One cup of cocoa butter (chopped)

Method:

1. Heat the oven at 175 degrees Celsius. Use a cooking spray for greasing a baking dish.

2. Combine all the ingredients in a large bowl using a hand mixer.

3. Pour the mixture in the greased dish.

4. Bake for thirty minutes.

5. Cool the blondies and refrigerate for about three hours.

6. Cut the blondies in squares and serve.

Low Carb Ice Cream

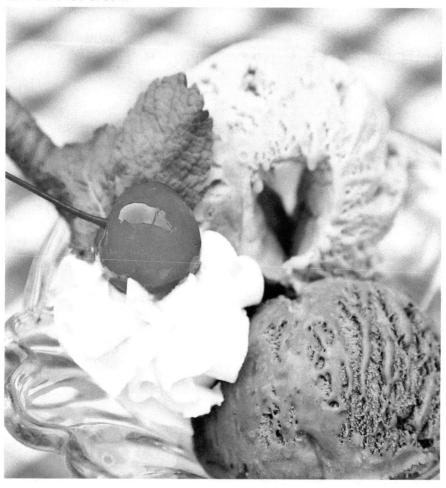

Total Prep & Cooking Time: Five hours and thirty-five minutes

Yields: Eight servings

Nutrition Facts: Calories: 337 | Protein: 2.2g | Carbs: 3.1g | Fat: 34g | Fiber: 0.3g

Ingredients

- Three tbsps. of butter
- Three cups of heavy cream
- One-third cup of powdered allulose
- One-fourth cup of coconut oil
- One tsp. of vanilla extract
- One medium-sized bean of vanilla

Method:

1. Take a pan and heat it over medium flame. Melt butter in it. Add a two-third cup of the heavy cream along with sweetener. Boil the mixture and simmer for thirty minutes.

2. Pour the mixture in a bowl and let it cool at room temperature. Add vanilla seeds from the bean along with the vanilla extract. Add coconut oil and mix well.

3. Add the remaining cream and combine until smooth.

4. Pour the mixture in a container and use a spatula for smoothening the top.

5. Freeze the ice cream for five hours. Ensure that you stir the ice cream mixture after every thirty minutes for the first two hours and then after every sixty minutes.

Chocolate Donut

Total Prep & Cooking Time: One hour and twenty-five minutes

Yields: Ten servings

Nutrition Facts: Calories: 219 | Protein: 5.1g | Carbs: 7.6g | Fat: 18.6g | Fiber: 3.1g

Ingredients

- Four eggs
- Half cup of butter (melted)
- Three tbsps. of milk
- One tsp. of stevia
- One-fourth cup of each
  - Coconut flour
  - Cocoa powder (unsweetened)
  - Sea salt
  - Baking soda

For the glaze:

- One tbsp. of avocado oil
- Three-fourth cup of chocolate chips

Method:

1. Heat the oven at 175 degrees Celsius.

2. Use a cooking spray for greasing donut pan of ten cavities.

3. Mix melted butter, eggs, and stevia, and milk in a bowl.

4. Add cocoa powder, coconut flour, baking soda, and salt.

5. Pour the mixture in the donut pan. Bake the donuts for fifteen minutes until set.

6. Let the donuts cool for fifteen minutes.

7. Add the chocolate chips in a bowl and melt in the microwave. Add avocado oil and stir.

8. Take out the donuts and dip them in the chocolate glaze.

9. Let the donuts sit for thirty minutes.

Chapter 4: Savory Recipes

In this section, I have included some tasty savory keto recipes that you can enjoy at any time of the day. So, let's have a look at them.

Keto McMuffin

Total Prep & Cooking Time: Twenty minutes

Yields: Two servings

Nutrition Facts: Calories: 610 | Protein: 24g | Carbs: 3.2g | Fat: 51.8g | Fiber: 6.9g

Ingredients

- One-fourth cup of each
    o Almond flour
    o Flaxmeal
- One-fourth tsp. of baking soda
- One egg
- Two tbsps. of heavy whipping cream
- One cup of cheddar cheese (shredded)
- Three tbsps. of water
- Salt (for seasoning)

For the filling:

- Two large eggs
- One tbsp. of butter
- Two cheddar cheese slices
- One tsp. of Dijon mustard
- Pepper and salt (for seasoning)

Method:

1. Combine all the dry ingredients. Mix well.

2. Add cream, water, and egg. Combine well using a fork.

3. Add the shredded cheese and mix.

4. Pour the mixture in greased ramekins. Microwave the mixture at high settings for two minutes.

5. Take a pan and fry the eggs. Add pepper and salt for seasoning.

6. Cut the prepared muffins in half. Spread butter on the inside portion of the muffin halves.

7. Top the muffin slices with egg, cheese, and mustard.

8. Serve immediately.

Sausage Hash With Rainbow Chard

Total Prep & Cooking Time: Twenty-five minutes

Yields: Two servings

Nutrition Facts: Calories: 570 | Protein: 25g | Carbs: 7.6g | Fat: 44.6g | Fiber: 5.6g

Ingredients

- Two-hundred grams of Swiss chard
- Two cups of cauliflower rice
- One-hundred and fifty grams of sausage meat
- Three tbsps. of lard
- Two garlic cloves (chopped)
- One tbsp. of lemon juice
- One tsp. of Dijon mustard
- Pepper and salt
- Four poached eggs

Method:

1. Chop the chard stalks into small pieces.

2. Take a greased skillet and add the sausage meat. Cook for five minutes until browned. Keep aside

3. Add the remaining lard to the same skillet. Add the garlic. Cook for one minute and add the cauliflower rice. Cook the mixture for five minutes.

4. Add the chard and Dijon mustard. Combine well. Add lemon juice and cook the mixture for two minutes. Add pepper and salt for seasoning.

5. Add the sausage meat and mix.

6. Serve with poached eggs.

Veggie and Chicken Sausage Skillet
Total Prep & Cooking Time: Thirty minutes

Yields: Four servings

Nutrition Facts: Calories: 310 | Protein: 21g | Carbs: 9.3g | Fat: 22.3g | Fiber: 2.4g

Ingredients

- Three tbsps. of butter
- Five links of chicken sausage (sliced)
- Two garlic cloves (minced)
- One red onion (cut in chunks)
- One zucchini (sliced in rounds)
- One summer squash (sliced in rounds)
- One red capsicum (cut in chunks)
- One yellow capsicum (cut in chunks)
- Six cremini mushrooms (quartered)
- Half tsp. of each
  o Red pepper flakes (crushed)
  o Italian seasoning
- Pepper and salt

Method:

1. Take an iron skillet and melt some butter in it.

2. Add the sausage, onion, and garlic. Sauté the mixture for ten minutes.

3. Add the veggies and mix well. Add pepper flakes, Italian seasoning, pepper, and salt.

4. Sauté the mixture for fifteen minutes and serve hot.

Cheese and Crispy Salami

Total Prep & Cooking Time: Twenty-five minutes

Yields: Ten servings

Nutrition Facts: Calories: 37 | Protein: 2.3g | Carbs: 1.3g | Fat: 2.7g | Fiber: 6.3g

Ingredients

- Two ounces of dried salami
- One ounce of cream cheese
- Half cup of parsley (chopped)

Method:

1. Heat the oven at 170 degrees Celsius.

2. Slice the salami into thirty slices of a quarter inch.

3. Arrange the salami on a baking pan.

4. Bake them for fifteen minutes.

5. Top the salami with cream cheese along with parsley.

Buffalo Chicken Sandwich

Total Prep & Cooking Time: Twenty-five minutes

Yields: Four servings

Nutrition Facts: Calories: 480 | Protein: 27g | Carbs: 5.1g | Fat: 30g | Fiber: 2.2g

Ingredients

- Two cups of cooked chicken (shredded)
- One-third cup of red pepper sauce
- Three tbsps. of butter
- One-fourth tsp. of each
    o Celery seed spice
    o Sea salt
    o Garlic powder
- Two tbsps. of each
    o Blue cheese crumbles
    o Celery (minced)
- Four tbsps. of ranch dressing
- Three tbsps. of mayonnaise
- Four sandwich buns

Method:

1. Take a medium saucepan and melt butter in it. Add celery seed spice, red pepper sauce, sea salt, and garlic powder. Stir well.

2. Add the chicken along with celery to the pan. Mix well and cook for two minutes.

3. Add the mayonnaise and combine.

4. Cut the buns in half. Add half cup of prepared chicken mixture on the buns. Top the chicken with one tbsp. of ranch dressing and half tbsp. of cheese crumbles.

5. Place the other halves on top and serve.

Cream Cheese and Salmon Bites

Total Prep & Cooking Time: Twenty minutes

Yields: Ten servings

Nutrition Facts: Calories: 43 | Protein: 1.3g | Carbs: 0.3g | Fat: 4.6g | Fiber: 0.6g

Ingredients

- Two eggs
- Half cup of cream
- One tbsp. of salt
- One cup of cheese (shredded)
- One-third tsp. of dill (dried)
- One-third cup of cream cheese (diced)
- Two cups of salmon (smoked, chopped)

Method:

1. Combine cream, eggs, and salt in a bowl.

2. Add cheese, cream cheese, and dill. Mix well.

3. Grease a muffin tray with butter.

4. Pour the mixture in the muffin tray. Add some pieces of salmon into each muffin.

5. Bake the mixture in the oven for twenty minutes at 180 degrees Celsius.

6. Remove the bites and serve warm.Vegetable Turkey Pesto Bolognese

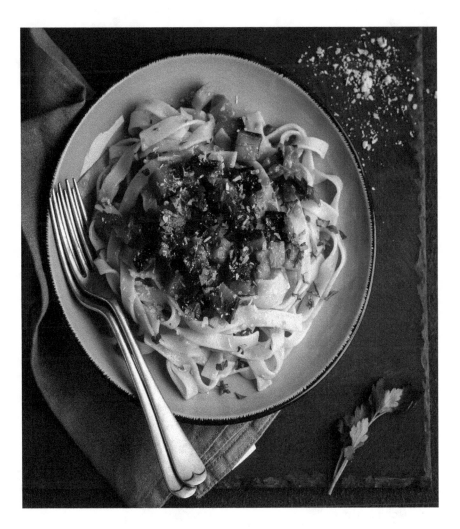

Total Prep & Cooking Time: Thirty minutes

Yields: Four servings

Nutrition Facts: Calories: 270 | Protein: 20.1g | Carbs: 4.3g | Fat: 13.2g | Fiber:
1.6g

Ingredients

- Two tsps. of oil

- One pound of turkey (ground)

- One cup of onion (diced)

- Two cups of each
    - Mushrooms (sliced)
    - Zucchini (sliced)

- Three tbsps. of pesto sauce

- Pasta of your choice (cooked)

- Grated cheese

Method:

1. Take a large skillet and add some oil. Add the turkey and cook until browned. Keep aside.

2. Add onions in the same and cook for two minutes. Add mushrooms and zucchini. Mix well.

3. Add the cooked turkey and combine it. Add pesto sauce simmer for five minutes.

4. Add cooked pasta along with cheese. Stir to combine. Simmer for two minutes.

5. Serve hot.

Turkey Patties

Total Prep & Cooking Time: Thirty minutes

Yields: Four servings

Nutrition Facts: Calories: 435 | Protein: 24g | Carbs: 4.5g | Fat: 37.2g | Fiber: 2.5g

Ingredients

- Five-hundred grams of ground turkey
- Half cup of almond flour
- One hot chili pepper (finely chopped)
- Two tsps. of Dijon mustard
- Two tbsps. of each
  - Parsley (chopped)
  - Lemon juice
  - Basil (chopped)
- Half tsp. of sea salt
- One tsp. black pepper (ground)
- Two spring onions (sliced finely)
- Two tbsps. of lard
- One egg
- Two garlic cloves (crushed)

Method:

1. Combine turkey, eggs, almond flour, garlic, pepper, lemon juice, Dijon mustard, basil, parsley, black pepper, and salt. Add the spring onions and mix well.

2. Make small patties using your hands.

3. Heat lard in a pan and add the patties. Cook the patties for five minutes on each side.

4. Let the patties sit for two minutes. Serve warm with spring onions.

Chapter 5: Poultry and Meat Recipes

Meat and poultry are rich in protein and various other nutrients that you need for perfect health. In this section, you will find some tasty poultry and meat keto recipes that you can make at home.

Beef Cabbage Skillet

Total Prep & Cooking Time: Thirty minutes

Yields: Four servings

Nutrition Facts: Calories: 357 | Protein: 13g | Carbs: 27g | Fat: 7.2g | Fiber: 11.3g

Ingredients

- Half green cabbage (shredded)
- Two tbsps. of butter
- One pound of beef (ground)
- Three tbsps. of taco seasoning
- One tsp. of minced onion (dried)
- One and a half cup of Mexican cheese blend
- Pepper and salt (according to taste)

Method:

1. Take a large skillet and heat one tbsp. of butter in it. Add shredded cabbage and sauté for two minutes. Keep aside.

2. Add one tbsp. of butter in the same skillet. Add the beef. Add onion, taco seasoning, and mix well. Cook for five minutes. Add one-fourth cup of water. Add the cooked cabbage along with pepper and salt. Combine half a cup of cheese.

3. Top with leftover cheese and place the skillet in the oven. Bake for ten minutes or until the cheese melts.

Meatball Casserole

Total Prep & Cooking Time: Three hours and thirty minutes

Yields: Six servings

Nutrition Facts: Calories: 470 | Protein: 37g | Carbs: 5.4g | Fat: 33.2g | Fiber: 4.7g

Ingredients

- Two pounds of beef (ground)
- Half cup of each
  - Mozzarella cheese
  - Parmesan cheese
- Two tbsps. of coconut flour
- Two large eggs
- Three-fourth tsp. of each
  - Onion (minced)
  - Salt
- One-fourth tsp. of Italian seasoning
- Half tsp. of garlic powder
- Twenty ounce can of spaghetti sauce
- Two cups of mozzarella cheese
- One tsp. of dried basil

Method:

1. Mix the ingredients in a bowl except for the spaghetti sauce, basil, and two cups of mozzarella cheese.

2. Heat a skillet on medium flame. Add one-fourth inch of coconut oil in the skillet.

3. Scoop meatballs from the mixture and add them to the skillet.

4. Cook the meatballs for five minutes until browned.

5. Place the meatballs in the base of a crockpot.

6. Add spaghetti sauce from the top.

7. Cook the meatballs on high for three hours.

8. Take out the meatballs in a baking dish.

9. Sprinkle cheese from the top.

10. Broil the meatballs for three minutes until cheese melts.

Beef Taquitos

Total Prep & Cooking Time: Forty minutes

Yields: Six servings

Nutrition Facts: Calories: 229 | Protein: 15.7g | Carbs: 1.6g | Fat: 16.3g | Fiber: 0.3g

Ingredients

- One cup of each
    - Cheddar cheese (shredded)
    - Mozzarella cheese (shredded)
- Half cup of parmesan cheese (grated)
- Half pound of beef (ground)
- One-fourth cup of onion (minced)
- Half tsp. of each
    - Paprika
    - Chili powder
    - Salt
    - Onion powder
    - Garlic powder
- One tsp. of cumin
- One-fourth tsp. of pepper
- One-third cup of water

Method:

1. Mix chili powder, cumin, garlic powder, onion powder, pepper, salt in a cup, and some water.

2. Take a skillet and brown the beef along with the onion. Add the mixture over the beef and simmer for ten minutes.

3. Mix all the cheese in a bowl. Divide the mixture of cheese for making six balls. Use parchment paper to line a baking sheet. Place them on the sheet and bake for eight minutes.

4. Let the cheese sheets cool down for two minutes.

5. Take one spoon of the beef mixture and place it on the edge of the cheese sheets. Repeat for the remaining sheets.

6. Roll them tightly for making cigar shape.

7. Serve warm.

Chicken Wings

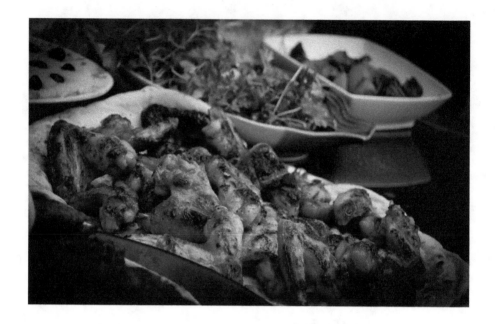

Total Prep & Cooking Time: Fifty minutes

Yields: Four servings

Nutrition Facts: Calories: 287 | Protein: 2.3g | Carbs: 12g | Fat: 16.3g | Fiber: 1.9g

Ingredients

- Two pounds of chicken wings
- Two tsps. of salt
- Three-fourth cup of coconut aminos
- One-fourth tsp. of each

- o Onion powder
- o Ginger (ground)
- o Garlic powder
- o Chili flakes

Method:

1. Place the wings on a baking tray.

2. Sprinkle some salt evenly on the wings.

3. Bake the chicken wings in the oven for forty minutes at 180 degrees Celsius.

4. Take a skillet and add coconut aminos. Add garlic powder, ginger, onion powder, and chili flakes. Simmer the sauce and stir until the sauce thickens.

5. Place the cooked wings in a large bowl and pour the sauce over the wings. Toss the cooked wings in the prepared sauce. Coat evenly.

6. Serve hot.

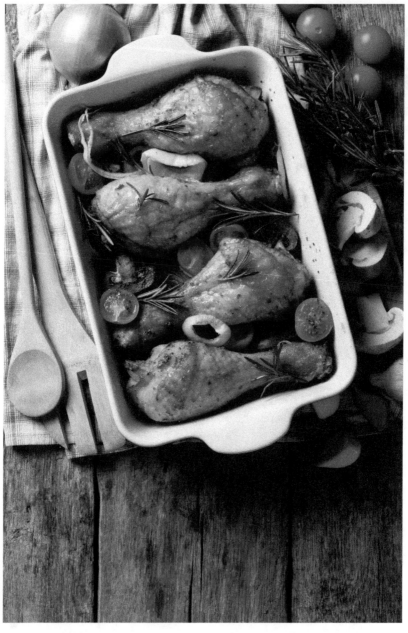

Total Prep & Cooking Time: One hour and ten minutes

Yields: Four servings

Nutrition Facts: Calories: 687 | Protein: 27.9g | Carbs: 10.1g | Fat: 58.9g | Fiber: 6g

Ingredients

- Four legs of chicken
- Four tbsps. of olive oil
- Two tbsps. of Italian seasoning
- Pepper and salt
- Twenty ounces of each
    o Cherry tomatoes
    o Broccoli

For the garlic butter:

- Four ounces of butter
- Two cloves of garlic (smashed)
- Pepper and salt

Method:

1. Toss the legs of the chicken with seasoning and oil.

2. Place the chicken legs in a baking sheet along with the tomatoes. Bake for forty-five minutes at 150 degrees Celsius.

3. As the chicken is cooking, cut the broccoli. Divide the florets and also slice the stem. Boil them in water for five minutes, along with some salt. Drain the broccoli water.

4. For making the garlic butter, combine all the ingredients in a small bowl.

5. Serve the cooked chicken legs with tomatoes, broccoli, and garlic butter by the side.

Note: Place the chicken legs in the oven with the skin side up.

Chapter 6: Staple Recipes

In this section, I have included some simple keto recipes made from everyday staples. Let's have a look at them.

Keto Waffles

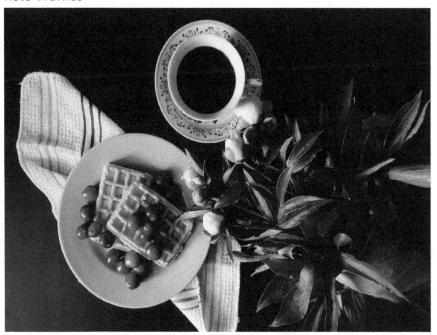

Total Prep & Cooking Time: Ten minutes

Yields: Two servings

Nutrition Facts: Calories: 160 | Protein: 21.3g | Carbs: 12.6g | Fat: 5.6g | Fiber: 10.3g

Ingredients

- Four tbsps. of coconut flour
- One tbsp. of each
    - Granulated sweetener
    - Apple sauce (unsweetened)
- One-fourth tsp. of each
    - Baking powder
    - Cinnamon
- Two-third cup of egg whites
- One-fourth cup of milk
- Half tsp. of vanilla extract
- One tsp. of coconut oil

Method:

1. Take a mixing bowl and mix the dry ingredients. Keep aside.

2. Add egg whites, vanilla extract, milk, and apple sauce in a bowl. Pour this mixture into the mixture of dry ingredients. Mix well.

3. Heat a waffle iron and grease with cooking spray or oil.

4. Add the waffle batter and cook for five minutes until fluffy and crisp.

Cookie Dough

Total Prep & Cooking Time: Ten minutes

Yields: Four servings

Nutrition Facts: Calories: 130 | Protein: 4.6g | Carbs: 4.3g | Fat: 12g | Fiber: 2.9g

Ingredients

- Half cup of almond flour
- Two tbsps. of each
    - Sticky sweetener
    - Granulated sweetener
    - Coconut flour
- One and a half tbsp. of coconut oil
- One tbsp. of chocolate chips

Method:

1. Combine coconut flour, almond flour, and granulated sugar in a bowl.

2. Add coconut oil and sticky sweetener. Mix well. Add the chocolate chips.

3. You can either enjoy the dough immediately or refrigerate it for thirty minutes.

Baked Tofu

Total Prep & Cooking Time: One hour and ten minutes

Yields: Two servings

Nutrition Facts: Calories: 131.3 | Protein: 11.3g | Carbs: 3.1g | Fat: 8.6g | Fiber: 1.7g

Ingredients

- One block of tofu (firm)
- One tbsp. of each
  - Soy sauce
  - Sesame oil
  - Tamari
- Half tsp. of each
  - Ginger
  - Garlic powder
  - Cayenne powder

Method:

1. Mix all the listed ingredients except for the tofu. Let the marinade sit for five minutes.

2. Chop the block of tofu into small pieces. Add the tofu cubes in the marinade. Refrigerate for half an hour.

3. Use parchment paper for lining a baking tray. Add the marinated tofu and bake for thirty minutes. Flip the tofu cubes halfway.

4. Serve immediately.

Cauliflower Fried Rice

Total Prep & Cooking Time: Twenty minutes

Yields: Four servings

Nutrition Facts: Calories: 135 | Protein: 7.9g | Carbs: 10.3g | Fat: 7.6g | Fiber: 8.6g

Ingredients

- Two tbsps. of sesame oil
- Two garlic cloves (finely chopped)
- One onion (finely chopped)
- Two scallions
- One-fourth cup of carrots (finely chopped)
- Eight cups of cauliflower rice
- Half cup of soy sauce
- One-fourth tsp. of cayenne pepper

Method:

1. Take a large wok and heat it over a medium flame. Addsome oil in it. Add garlic and onion. Cook for two minutes. Add scallions and carrots. Sauté for two minutes.

2. Add the cauliflower rice and combine well. Add cayenne and soy sauce. Fry for four minutes.

3. Serve the fried rice with scallions from the top.

PART III

Vegan Keto

The ketogenic diet is a popular diet that is low in carbohydrates and is high in fat. The diet involves moderate consumption of protein that can promote weight loss and can also help in the improvement of overall health. Although the keto diet is mostly associated with animal-based foods, it can also be adapted for fitting food items that are plant-based, specifically vegan diets. The vegan diet does not include any kind of animal product. But, with proper planning, even vegans can enjoy the benefits of the keto diet.

In keto diet, carbs are reduced to 45-50 grams per day for maintaining and reaching ketosis. Ketosis is a metabolic process of the body for burning fat as fuel in place of glucose. People who follow a vegan keto diet rely on plant-based foods such as grains, veggies, and fruits. As the requirement of fat is more, plant-based food products such as avocados, coconut oil, nuts, and seeds are included in the vegan keto diet. Vegan keto diet comes along with various benefits. It can reduce the overall risk of developing severe health conditions like diabetes, heart diseases, and specific cancers. For instance, studies revealed that all those who follow vegan keto diet have a 74% lower risk of high blood pressure and a 75% risk reduction for type 2 diabetes.

It has also been found that people who follow a vegan keto diet can lose more weight than those who eat animal-based food products. The vegan keto diet can also increase the level of adiponectin, a protein responsible for regulating blood sugar and fat metabolism. When the level of adiponectin is high, it can help in the reduction of inflammation, better control over blood sugar, and can also help in reducing diseases related to obesity. Keto diet has also shown evident results in reducing the risk factors of heart diseases, along with LDL cholesterol, blood pressure, and high triglycerides. Combining a vegan diet along with a ketogenic diet can effectively impact your overall health.

When you start following a vegan diet, you will need to reduce the intake of carbs and replace them with healthy fats. You will also need to include vegan high protein sources. You cannot consume animal-based products such as poultry, egg, meat, seafood, and dairy. Here are some examples of the food items that you will need to avoid altogether:

- **Dairy:** Butter, milk, yogurt

- **Poultry and meat:** Turkey, pork, beef, chicken

- **Egg:** Egg yolk and egg white

- **Animal-based items:** Whey protein, egg white protein, honey

- **Seafood:** Shrimp, fish, mussels, clams

Here are some examples of the food items that you will need to reduce:

- **Sugar-based drinks:** Soda, juice, sweet tea, sports drinks, smoothies

- **Starches and grains:** Bread, cereal, pasta, baked items

- **Starchy veggies:** Sweet potatoes, potatoes, beet, squash, peas

Turn to the next page for recipes that can help you get started with a vegan keto diet.

Chapter 1: Breakfast Recipes

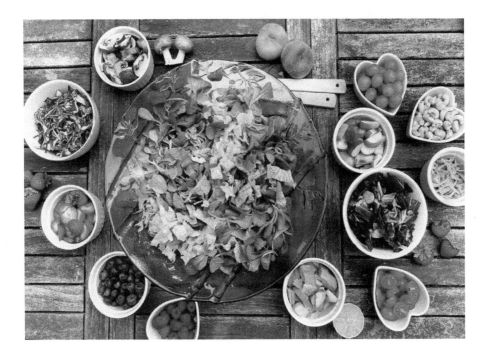

Breakfast is an important part of any diet plan. Here are some tasty vegan keto recipes for you.

Tofu Scramble

Total Prep & Cooking Time: Twenty minutes

Yields: Two servings

Nutrition Facts: Calories: 204 | Protein: 21.3g | Carbs: 3.6g | Fat: 12.3g | Fiber: 0.8g

Ingredients:

- Two-hundred grams of tofu (firm)
- One tbsp. of vegan butter
- Two tbsps. of nutritional yeast
- Half tsp. of each
  - Paprika
  - Turmeric
  - Garlic powder
- One tsp. of Dijon mustard
- One-fourth tsp. of each
  - Onion powder
  - Black salt
- One-third cup of soy milk

Method:

1. Place tofu in a bowl. Use a fork for mashing the tofu. Leave some medium-sized chunks.

2. Add turmeric, yeast, paprika, garlic powder, Dijon mustard, onion powder, and black salt in a bowl. Combine the ingredients. Add soy milk and whisk properly for making a smooth sauce.

3. Add vegan butter to a medium pan. Add mashed tofu and fry it for two minutes until browned. Add prepared sauce to the mashed tofu. Combine well. Cook for five minutes until the sauce gets absorbed by the tofu.

4. Serve hot.

Low Carb Pancakes

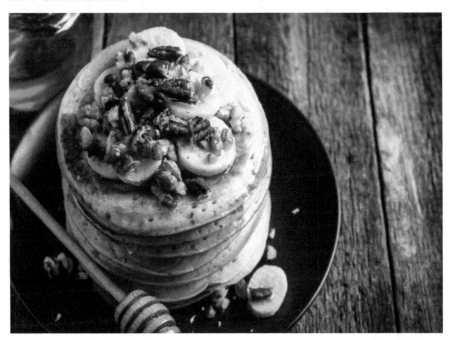

Total Prep & Cooking Time: Thirty minutes

Yields: Two servings

Nutrition Facts: Calories: 249 | Protein: 10.4g | Carbs: 12.8g | Fat: 19.6g | Fiber: 9.8g

Ingredients:

- Two tbsps. of almond butter
- One-fourth cup of almond milk (unsweetened)

- One tbsp. of coconut flour
- One and a half tbsps. of ground flax
- Half tsp. of baking powder

Method:

1. Take a small bowl and combine the almond milk with almond butter.

2. Take another bowl and combine the dry ingredients.

3. Add the mixture of milk to the dry mixture. Combine well. Allow the batter to sit for five minutes.

4. Heat a skillet over medium flame.

5. Add one spoon of batter to the warm skillet. Evenly spread out the batter—Cook the pancakes for five minutes on each side. Repeat the same for the remaining batter.

6. Serve the pancakes hot with almond butter from the top.

Cauliflower Hashbrowns

Total Prep & Cooking Time: Fifty minutes

Yields: Six servings

Nutrition Facts: Calories: 142 | Protein: 6.3g | Carbs: 18.2g | Fat: 5.6g | Fiber: 4.3g

Ingredients:

- Half head of cauliflower (separate the florets)
- One tbsp. of coconut oil
- Half onion (chopped)
- One-fourth cup of chickpea flour
- One tbsp. of cornstarch
- Half tsp. of each
  - Salt
  - Garlic powder
- Two tbsps. of water

Method:

1. Preheat your oven at 200 degrees Celsius; use parchment paper for lining a baking sheet. Spray the parchment paper with some oil.

2. Add onion and cauliflower in a blender and blend until crumbly.

3. Combine chickpea flour, cornstarch, salt, garlic powder, and water in a bowl. Mix well.

4. Add the cauliflower crumbles to the batter. Combine properly.

5. Shape the hashbrowns into thick patties.

6. Bake the hashbrowns in the oven for forty minutes. Flip the patties halfway.

7. Serve hot.

Vanilla Waffles

Total Prep & Cooking Time: Twenty minutes

Yields: Two servings

Nutrition Facts: Calories: 160 | Protein: 21.3g | Carbs: 13.6g | Fat: 4.9g | Fiber: 9.9g

Ingredients:

- One-fourth cup of oat flour
- Half scoop of protein powder (vanilla)
- One tbsp. of each
    - Flaxseed (ground)
    - Granulated sweetener of your choice
- One-fourth tsp. of baking powder
- Half cup of almond milk
- One-fourth tsp. of vanilla extract

Method:

1. Add the dry ingredients in a large bowl. Combine well.

2. Add baking powder, flaxseed, vanilla extract, and one-fourth cup of the almond milk in a bowl. Whisk well and allow it to sit for four minutes.

3. Add the dry ingredients to the mixture of vanilla extract. Combine properly.

4. Heat up a waffle iron and add two spoons of waffle mixture.

5. Cook for four minutes.

6. Serve hot.

Pecan And Cinnamon Porridge

Total Prep & Cooking Time: Twenty minutes

Yields: Two servings

Nutrition Facts: Calories: 580 | Protein: 13.4g | Carbs: 5.1g | Fat: 49.7g | Fiber: 10.8g

Ingredients:

- One-fourth cup of coconut milk
- One cup of almond butter
- Three-fourth cup of almond milk
- One tbsp. of coconut oil
- Two tbsps. of chia seeds
- Three tbsps. of hemp seeds
- One-fourth cup of each
  - Pecans
  - Flaked coconut
- Half tsp. of cinnamon

Method:

1. Mix almond milk, coconut milk, coconut oil, and almond butter in a pan. Simmer the mixture over a medium flame.

2. Once the mixture gets hot, remove from heat.

3. Add hemp seeds, chia seeds, pecans, and coconut flakes. Combine the ingredients and add cinnamon. Allow the porridge to sit for ten minutes.

4. Serve cold or hot with coconut flakes from the top.

Chapter 2: Appetizers Recipes

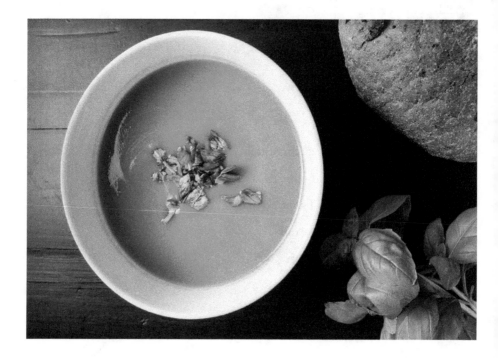

Appetizers play an important role in a complete meal. There are various vegan keto appetizers that you can include in your diet plan. Let's have a look at them.

Arugula Salad

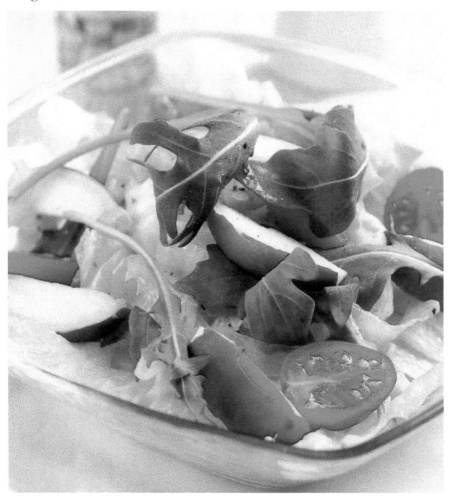

Total Prep & Cooking Time: Ten minutes

Yields: Two servings

Nutrition Facts: Calories: 41 | Protein: 0.7g | Carbs: 2.6g | Fat: 3.1g | Fiber: 0.9g

Ingredients:

- Six tbsps. of olive oil (extra virgin)
- Two tbsps. of lemon juice
- Salt and pepper (according to taste)
- Four cups of arugula

Method:

1. Take a small-sized bowl and whisk together olive oil and lemon juice. Add pepper and salt.

2. Add the arugula in a large bowl and add the dressing from the top. Toss to combine.

Cauliflower Soup

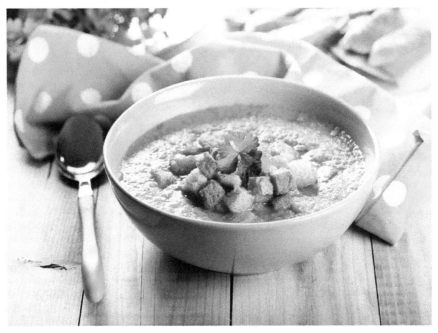

Total Prep & Cooking Time: Thirty minutes

Yields: Four servings

Nutrition Facts: Calories: 127 | Protein: 5.2g | Carbs: 15.6g | Fat: 5.6g | Fiber: 3.9g

Ingredients:

- One tbsp. of olive oil (extra virgin)
- One yellow onion (chopped)

- One garlic clove (minced)
- One cauliflower (florets separated)
- Six cups of vegetable stock
- Three sprigs of thyme
- One bay leaf
- Pepper and salt (to taste)
- One-fourth cup of vegan cream

Method:

1. Take a deep pot and heat oil in it. Add onions and cook it for six minutes until tender. Add minced garlic to the pot. Add the florets of cauliflower, thyme, vegetable stock, and bay leaf. Simmer the mixture for twenty minutes until the florets are tender.

2. Remove bay leaf along with thyme. Blend the mixture using a stick blender until smooth. Add vegan cream and simmer for five minutes.

3. Serve with olive oil from the top.

Cauliflower Zucchini Fritters

Total Prep & Cooking Time: Twenty minutes

Yields: Eight servings

Nutrition Facts: Calories: 53 | Protein: 4.2g | Carbs: 5.9g | Fat: 2.1g | Fiber: 3.6g

Ingredients:

- Half head of a cauliflower
- Two large zucchinis
- One-fourth cup of flour
- Half tsp. of salt
- One-fourth tsp. of black pepper (ground)

Method:

1. Add zucchini in a blender and grate.

2. Add the cauliflower to the food processor and blend into small chunks.

3. Put the veggies in a dishtowel and squeeze out as much water as possible.

4. Transfer the veggies to a bowl; add flour, pepper, and salt. Mix well.

5. Shape the mixture into small patties.

6. Heat oil in a pan. Add the patties to the pan—Cook for three minutes on all sides.

7. Serve hot with any dipping sauce of your choice.

Notes:

- You can add chickpeas for extra flavor.

- The leftover fritters can be stored in the fridge for two days.

Zucchini Noodles And Avocado Sauce

Total Prep & Cooking Time: Thirty minutes

Yields: Two servings

Nutrition Facts: Calories: 311 | Protein: 6.7g | Carbs: 17.8g | Fat: 24.5g | Fiber: 9.9g

Ingredients:

- One large zucchini
- Two cups of basil
- One-third cup of water
- Four tbsps. of pine nuts
- Two tbsps. of lemon juice
- One large avocado
- Twelve cherry tomatoes (sliced)

Method:

1. Start with the zucchini noodles. Use a peeler or a spiralizer for making the noodles. In case you do not have a peeler or spiralizer, use a sharp knife for cutting thin strips of zucchini.

2. Add all the ingredients in the food processor except for the cherry tomatoes.

3. Combine sauce, noodles, and cherry tomatoes in a bowl. Toss for combining.

4. Serve at room temperature, or you can also chill in the freezer for ten minutes.

Notes:

- You can add any fresh herbs and veggies that you want to. You can replace zucchini with other vegetables such as carrots, cabbage, beet, squash, etc.

- Pine nuts can be replaced with any nuts of your choice.

- You can store the leftover noodles in the fridge for two days.

Roasted Brussels Sprouts

Total Prep & Cooking Time: Thirty minutes

Yields: Four servings

Nutrition Facts: Calories: 130 | Protein: 3.8g | Carbs: 11.3g | Fat: 9.7g | Fiber: 4.6g

Ingredients:

- Four-hundred grams of Brussels sprouts (halved)
- Two tbsps. of olive oil
- Black pepper and salt (according to taste)

Method:

1. Preheat your oven to 220 degrees Celsius.

2. Take a large baking sheet. Spread the Brussels sprouts on the sheet. Drizzle olive oil from the top. Season with pepper and salt. Toss for combining.

3. Roast the sprouts in the oven for twenty-five minutes until all the are crispy outside and tender from inside.

4. Serve hot.

Chapter 3: Main Course Recipes

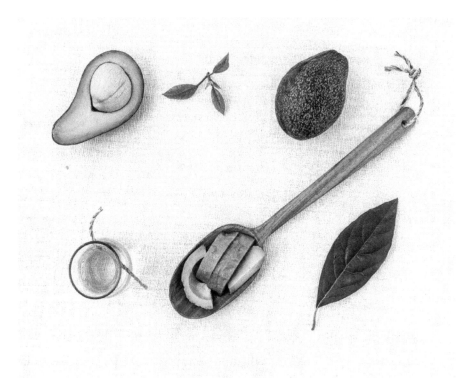

After you are done with the appetizers, now it is time to have a look at the main course recipes. I have included some tasty vegan keto main course recipes in this section that you can enjoy in your lunch and dinner as well.

Mushroom Tomato Spaghetti Squash

Total Prep & Cooking Time: Forty minutes

Yields: Four servings

Nutrition Facts: Calories: 240 | Protein: 6.3g | Carbs: 21.3g | Fat: 8.9g | Fiber:

8.6g

Ingredients:

- Six cups of spaghetti squash (cooked)
- Two cups of tomatoes (diced)
- Four garlic cloves (minced)
- Eight ounces of mushrooms (sliced)
- One-third cup of onions (chopped)
- One-fourth cup of pine nuts (toasted)
- A handful of basil
- Three tbsps. of olive oil
- Black pepper and salt (for seasoning)

Method:

1. Cook the spaghetti squash in the way you like. The easiest way to cook is by roasting in the oven. When the squash is cool enough, remove the seeds along with the stringy bits. Shred the squash with a fork. Keep aside.

2. Take a sauté pan and heat some oil in it. Add mushrooms and onions to the pan. Keep cooking for four minutes until onion turns translucent. Add minced garlic to the pan and cook for two minutes. Add tomatoes and keep stirring.

3. Add the cooked spaghetti squash to the mixture and toss it well for combining. Add pine nuts and basil—season with salt and black pepper.

4. Serve hot.

Vegan Shakshuka
Total Prep & Cooking Time: Twenty-five minutes

Yields: Two servings

Nutrition Facts: Calories: 274 | Protein: 21.3g | Carbs: 22.6g | Fat: 9.5g | Fiber: 9.7g

Ingredients:

- One tbsp. of olive oil
- Four garlic cloves
- One can of diced tomatoes
- Pepper and salt (according to taste)
- Two tsps. of dried herbs
- Half tsp. of chili flakes (dried)
- One medium-sized block of tofu
- Black salt (optional)

Method:

1. Take a large skillet and add olive in it. Heat the oil and add garlic to the skillet. Brown the garlic a bit.

2. Add diced tomatoes, pepper, salt, chili flakes, and dried herbs. Mix the ingredients properly and simmer for five minutes.

3. Cut the tofu block in rounds and add them to the skillet.

4. Lower the flame and simmer the shakshuka for fifteen minutes. Cook until the sauce thickens, and the tofu rounds are tender.

5. Sprinkle some black salt from the top.

6. Serve with crusty bread slices or toast by the side.

Zucchini Lasagna

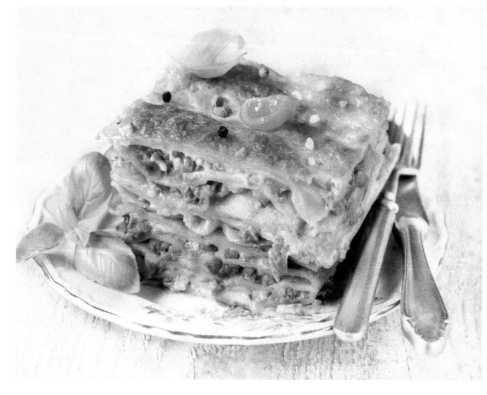

Total Prep & Cooking Time: One hour and twenty minutes

Yields: Eight servings

Nutrition Facts: Calories: 392 | Protein: 6.3g | Carbs: 18.7g | Fat: 33.9g | Fiber: 7.6g

Ingredients:

For vegan ricotta:

- Three cups of macadamia nuts (raw)
- Two tbsps. of nutritional yeast
- Half cup of basil (chopped)
- Two tsps. of oregano (dried)

- One medium-sized lemon (juiced)
- One tbsp. of olive oil (extra virgin)
- One tsp. of each
  - Black pepper
  - Salt
- One-third cup of water

Other ingredients:

- One jar of marinara sauce
- Three medium-sized zucchini squash (sliced thinly)

Method:

1. Preheat your oven at 160/175 degrees Celsius.

2. Add the nuts to a blender and blend. Scrape down the sides. Blend for making a fine meal.

3. Add yeast, oregano, basil, olive oil, lemon juice, pepper, water, and salt to the blended nuts in the blender. Blend for making a smooth paste.

4. Adjust the taste by adding seasonings. If you want more cheesiness, add yeast.

5. Pour one cup of marinara sauce in a baking dish. Line the dish with zucchini slices.

6. Add one scoop of ricotta mixture over the zucchini layer and spread evenly. Repeat for the remaining layers.

7. Cover the baking dish using foil and bake the lasagna for forty-five minutes. Remove the foil. Bake again for fifteen minutes.

8. Allow the lasagna to cool down for ten minutes.

9. Serve warm with basil from the top.

Arugula Tomato And Avocado Salad

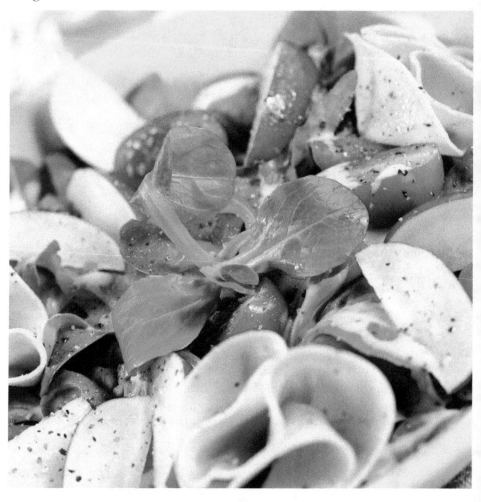

Total Prep & Cooking Time: Fifteen minutes

Yields: Four servings

Nutrition Facts: Calories: 259 | Protein: 4.2g | Carbs: 5.2g | Fat: 17g | Fiber: 0.9g

Ingredients:

- One cup of cherry tomatoes (halved)
- Half cup of yellow cherry tomatoes (halved)
- Five ounces of arugula (chopped)
- Two large avocados (cut in chunks)
- Half cup of red onion (diced)
- Six leaves of basil (sliced)

For vinaigrette:

- Two tbsps. of balsamic vinegar
- One tbsp. of each:
  - Maple syrup
  - Olive oil
  - Lemon juice
- One clove of garlic (minced)
- Half tsp. of Italian seasoning
- One-fourth tsp. of each:
  - Pepper
  - Sea salt

Method:

1. Combine tomatoes, arugula, basil, red onion, and chunks of avocado in a mixing bowl.

2. Whisk together olive oil, lemon juice, vinegar, maple syrup, garlic, pepper, salt, and Italian seasoning in a small bowl. Mix well.

3. Add the dressing to the salad mix. Toss well for combining.

4. Serve with basil from the top.

Mushroom Fried Rice

Total Prep & Cooking Time: Thirty minutes

Yields: Six servings

Nutrition Facts: Calories: 118 | Protein: 10.2g | Carbs: 14.9g | Fat: 2.8g | Fiber: 7.3g

Ingredients:

- Four tbsps. of water
- One onion (diced)
- Two-inch piece of ginger (grated)
- Three cloves of garlic (minced)
- Ten ounces mix of veggies (carrots, peas, and edamame)
- Two cups of mushrooms (shitake)
- Four cups of cauliflower rice
- Three tbsps. of tamari
- Half tsp. of sesame oil
- One-fourth cup of green onion (sliced)

Method:

1. Take a large pan and add water to it. Sauté the onions in water for four minutes until translucent and soft; add ginger and garlic to the pan. Stir and cook the mixture for three minutes.

2. Add a mixture of veggies to the pan along with the mushrooms. Stir well for combining. Add the cauliflower rice and mix well. Let the fried rice cook for fifteen minutes until the water dissolves.

3. Add half tsp. of sesame oil and three tsps. of tamari. Stir again.

4. Serve hot with green onions from the top.

Note: You can store the leftover fried rice in the fridge for one day.

Chapter 4: Snacks And Dessert Recipes

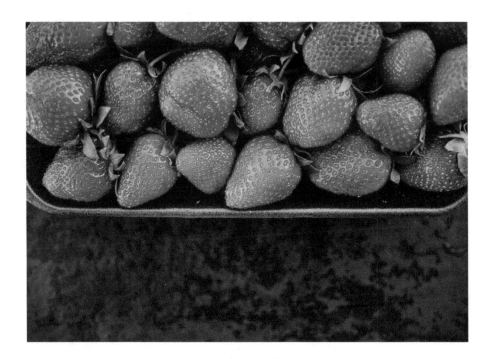

Everyone loves to have some snacks in between their meals and a good dessert after having a sumptuous meal. So, I have included some tasty and easy snacks and dessert recipes in this section that you can include in your vegan keto diet.

Almond Flour Crackers

Total Prep & Cooking Time: Twenty-five minutes

Yields: Six servings

Nutrition Facts: Calories: 149 | Protein: 4.2g | Carbs: 5.7g | Fat: 12.3g | Fiber: 3.2g

Ingredients:

- One cup of almond flour
- Two tbsps. of sunflower seeds
- One tbsp. of flax meal or psyllium husks
- Three-fourth tsp. of sea salt
- Three tbsps. of water
- One tbsp. of coconut oil

Method:

1. Preheat your oven at 160/175 degrees Celsius.

2. Add sunflower seeds, almond flour, sea salt, and flax meal in a food processor. Process the ingredients.

3. Add the coconut oil along with water to the mixture and pulse again. Blend until a dough forms.

4. Add the dough on parchment paper and flatten the dough using your hands. Cover the cracker dough using another parchment paper and flatten with the help of a rolling pin.

5. Remove the upper layer sheet of parchment paper. Cut the dough into several crackers into the size and shape that you want.

6. Sprinkle some sea salt from the top.

7. Bake the crackers for fifteen minutes at 175 degrees Celsius until the edges are crisp and brown.

Guacamole

Total Prep & Cooking Time: Twenty minutes

Yields: Four servings

Nutrition Facts: Calories: 180.2 | Protein: 2.3g | Carbs: 12.1g | Fat: 15.2g | Fiber: 7.9g

Ingredients:

- Three ripe avocados
- Half onion (diced)
- Two tomatoes (diced)
- Three tbsps. of cilantro (chopped)
- One jalapeno pepper (diced)
- Two cloves of garlic (minced)
- One lime (juiced)
- Half tsp. of sea salt

Method:

1. Slice the avocado and remove the pit. Skin them and place them in a bowl.

2. Use a fork for mashing the avocados. You can either make it smooth or chunky.

3. Add remaining ingredients and mix well.

4. Serve with crackers.

Strawberry And Avocado Ices

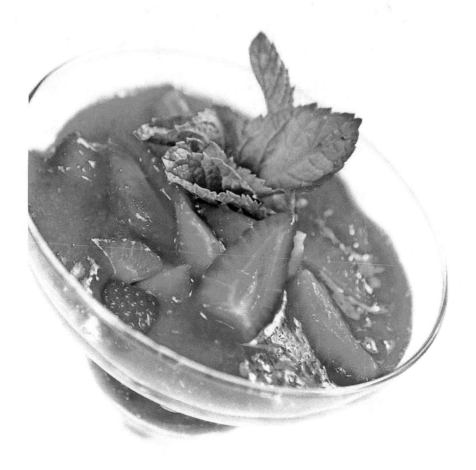

Total Prep & Cooking Time: One hour and ten minutes

Yields: Four servings

Nutrition Facts: Calories: 93 | Protein: 3.1g | Carbs: 4.2g | Fat: 7.2g | Fiber: 4g

Ingredients:

- Two-hundred grams of strawberries (chopped)
- One avocado (chopped)
- Two tsps. of balsamic vinegar
- Half tsp. of vanilla extract
- Two tsps. of maple syrup

Method:

1. Add avocado, strawberries, vanilla, and vinegar in a bowl. Use a hand blender for pulsing the mixture. You can also use a food processor. Blend for reaching the consistency that you want. Add maple syrup and mix again.

2. Pour the mixture into small containers and add strawberry slices from the top. Cover the containers using a plastic wrap.

3. Freeze the containers for one hour.

4. Allow the containers to sit at room temperature for five minutes before serving.

Chocolate And Peanut Butter Ice Cream

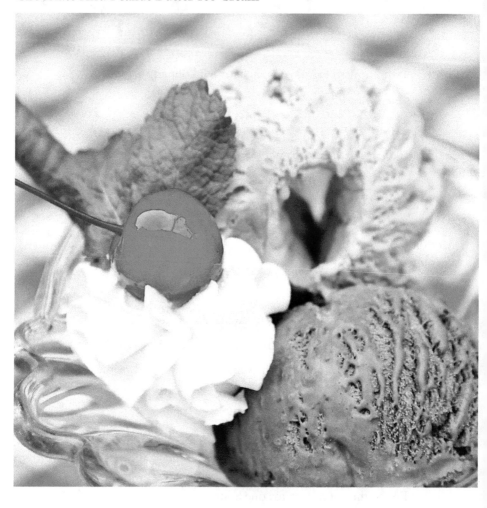

Total Prep & Cooking Time: Three hours and ten minutes

Yields: Six servings

Nutrition Facts: Calories: 360 | Protein: 5.8g | Carbs: 7.9g | Fat: 34g | Fiber: 4.2g

Ingredients:

- One can of coconut milk
- Half cup of each
    - Powdered sweetener of your choice
    - Peanut butter
- One-third cup of coconut oil
- One-fourth cup of cocoa powder
- One pinch of salt

Method:

1. Add the ingredients in a blender. Keep blending until smooth.

2. Pour the ice cream mixture in a glass container. Cover the container and freeze for half an hour.

3. Remove the cover and stir the mixture, especially from the sides right to the center. Cover again and freeze for thirty minutes. Stir the mixture once again and freeze for two hours.

4. Scoop the ice cream into serving bowls and garnish with peanut butter from the top.

Carrot Cake

Total Prep & Cooking Time: One hour

Yields: Six servings

Nutrition Facts: Calories: 150 | Protein: 3.1g | Carbs: 4.1g | Fat: 6.3g | Fiber: 3.2g

Ingredients:

- Two cups of flour
- One and a half cup of almond flour
- One-fourth tsp. of baking soda
- One tbsp. of cinnamon
- One tsp. of nutmeg
- One carrot (shredded)
- One-third cup of walnuts (chopped)
- Two tbsps. of shredded coconut
- Half tbsp. of apple cider vinegar
- Three-fourth cup of vegan milk (any vegan milk of your choice)
- Half cup of olive oil
- One-fourth cup of maple syrup

Method:

1. Start by preheating your oven at 180 degrees Celsius. Use parchment paper for lining a square baking pan.

2. Combine maple syrup, olive oil, milk of your choice, and vinegar in a bowl. Add walnuts, carrots, and coconut to the mixture. Mix well.

3. Add flour, almond flour, spices, and baking soda. Combine the ingredients.

4. Pour the prepared batter in the lined pan. Bake the mixture for half an hour.

5. Allow the cake to cool down for five minutes.

6. Serve warm with a frosting of your choice.

Notes:

- Before baking the cake, add some shredded carrots from the top for extra flavor. It will make the cake look beautiful, as well.

- In case you have any leftover cake, you can store it in the fridge for one day.

- You can use almond milk for the best results.

Almond And Chocolate Pudding

Total Prep & Cooking Time: Five hours and ten minutes Yields: Three servings

Nutrition Facts: Calories: 280 | Protein: 5.2g | Carbs: 11.7g | Fat: 24.6g | Fiber: 8.9g

Ingredients:

- Two cups of almond milk
- Half cup of coconut cream
- Three tbsps. of vegan sweetener (of your choice)
- One avocado (pitted)
- Three tbsps. of cocoa powder
- One tsp. of vanilla extract
- Two tsps. of almond extract
- Sliced almonds (to garnish)

Method:

1. Add the listed ingredients in a high-power food processor. Blend the ingredients until smooth.

2. Pour the mixture into serving cups. Cover the cups and refrigerate for about five hours.

3. Serve with sliced almonds from the top.

Notes:

- This pudding is gluten-free and is ketogenic as well.
- You can add chocolate chips from the top for extra flavor.
- You can store the leftover pudding in the fridge for two days.

PART IV

Smoothie Diet Recipes

The smoothie diet is all about replacing some of your meals with smoothies that are loaded with veggies and fruits. It has been found that the smoothie diet is very helpful in losing weight along with excess fat. The ingredients of the smoothies will vary, but they will focus mainly on vegetables and fruits. The best part about the smoothie diet is that there is no need to count your calorie intake and less food tracking. The diet is very low in calories and is also loaded with phytonutrients.

Apart from weight loss, there are various other benefits of the smoothie diet. It can help you to stay full for a longer time as most smoothies are rich in fiber. It can also help you to control your cravings as smoothies are full of flavor and nutrients. Whenever you feel like snacking, just prepare a smoothie, and you are good to go. Also, smoothies can aid in digestion as they are rich in important minerals and vitamins. Fruits such as mango are rich in carotenoids that can help in improving your skin quality. As the smoothie diet is mainly based on veggies and fruits, it can detoxify your body.

In this section, you will find various recipes of smoothies that you can include in your smoothie diet.

Chapter 1: Fruit Smoothies

The best way of having fruits is by making smoothies. Fruit smoothies can help you start your day with loads of nutrients so that you can remain energetic throughout the day. Here are some easy-to-make fruit smoothie recipes that you can enjoy during any time of the day.

Quick Fruit Smoothie

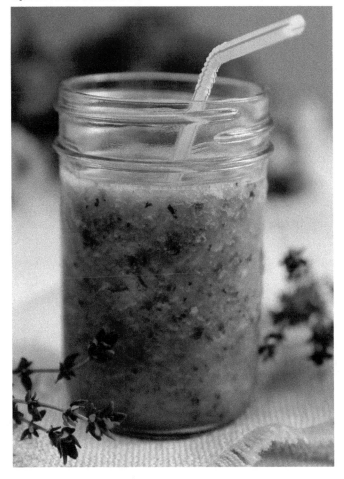

Total Prep & Cooking Time: Fifteen minutes

Yields: Four servings

Nutrition Facts: Calories: 115.2 | Protein: 1.2g | Carbs: 27.2g | Fat: 0.5g | Fiber: 3.6g

Ingredients

- One cup of strawberries
- One banana (cut in chunks)
- Two peaches
- Two cups of ice
- One cup of orange and mango juice

Method:

1. Add banana, strawberries, and peaches in a blender.

2. Blend until frothy and smooth.

3. Add the orange and mango juice and blend again. Add ice for adjusting the consistency and blend for two minutes.

4. Divide the smoothie in glasses and serve with mango chunks from the top.

Triple Threat Smoothie
Total Prep & Cooking Time: Ten minutes

Yields: Four servings

Nutrition Facts: Calories: 132.2 | Protein: 3.4g | Carbs: 27.6g | Fat: 1.3g | Fiber: 2.7g

Ingredients

- One kiwi (sliced)
- One banana (chopped)
- One cup of each
  - Ice cubes
  - Strawberries
- Half cup of blueberries
- One-third cup of orange juice
- Eight ounces of peach yogurt

Method:

1. Add kiwi, strawberries, and bananas in a food processor.

2. Blend until smooth.

3. Add the blueberries along with orange juice. Blend again for two minutes.

4. Add peach yogurt and ice cubes. Give it a pulse.

5. Pour the prepared smoothie in smoothie glasses and serve with blueberry chunks from the top.

Tropical Smoothie

Total Prep & Cooking Time: Fifteen minutes

Yields: Two servings

Nutrition Facts: Calories: 127.3 | Protein: 1.6g | Carbs: 30.5g | Fat: 0.7g | Fiber: 4.2g

Ingredients

- One mango (seeded)
- One papaya (cubed)
- Half cup of strawberries
- One-third cup of orange juice
- Five ice cubes

Method:

1. Add mango, strawberries, and papaya in a blender. Blend the ingredients until smooth.

2. Add ice cubes and orange juice for adjusting the consistency.

3. Blend again.

4. Serve with strawberry chunks from the top.

Fruit and Mint Smoothie

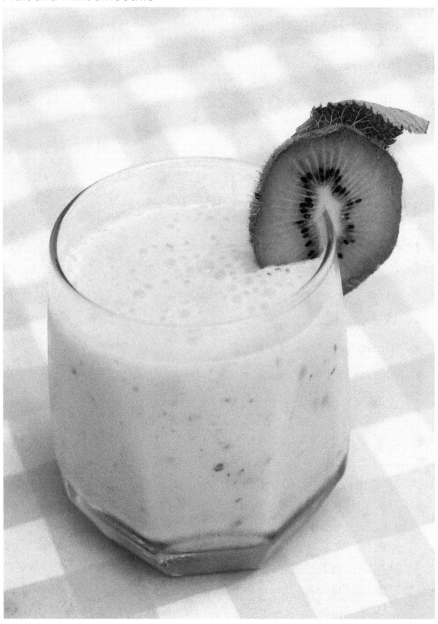

Total Prep & Cooking Time: Fifteen minutes

Yields: Two servings

Nutrition Facts: Calories: 90.3 | Protein: 0.7g | Carbs: 21.4g | Fat: 0.4g | Fiber: 2.5g

Ingredients

- One-fourth cup of each
    - o Applesauce (unsweetened)
    - o Red grapes (seedless, frozen)
- One tbsp. of lime juice
- Three strawberries (frozen)
- One cup of pineapple cubes
- Three mint leaves

Method:

1. Add grapes, lime juice, and applesauce in a blender. Blend the ingredients until frothy and smooth.

2. Add pineapple cubes, mint leaves, and frozen strawberries in the blender. Pulse the ingredients for a few times until the pineapple and strawberries are crushed.

3. Serve with mint leaves from the top.

Banana Smoothie

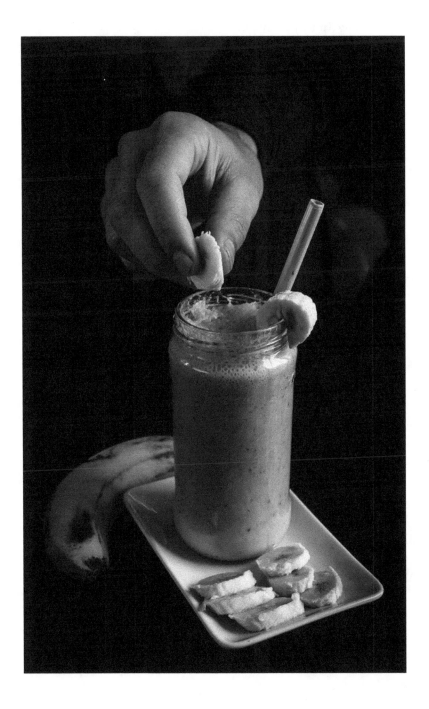

Total Prep & Cooking Time: Ten minutes

Yields: Four servings

Nutrition Facts: Calories: 122.6 | Protein: 1.3g | Carbs: 34.6g | Fat: 0.4g | Fiber: 2.2g

Ingredients

- Three bananas (sliced)
- One cup of fresh pineapple juice
- One tbsp. of honey
- Eight cubes of ice

Method:

1. Combine the bananas and pineapple juice in a blender.

2. Blend until smooth.

3. Add ice cubes along with honey.

4. Blend for two minutes.

5. Serve immediately.

Dragon Fruit Smoothie

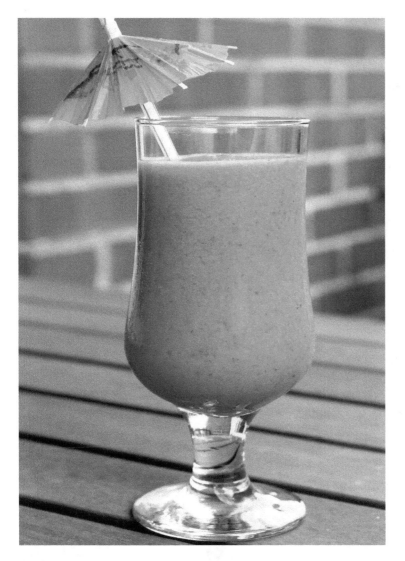

Total Prep & Cooking Time: Twenty minutes

Yields: Four servings

Nutrition Facts: Calories: 147.6 | Protein: 5.2g | Carbs: 21.4g | Fat: 6.4g | Fiber: 2.9g

Ingredients

- One-fourth cup of almonds
- Two tbsps. of shredded coconut
- One tsp. of chocolate chips
- One cup of yogurt
- One dragon fruit (chopped)
- Half cup of pineapple cubes
- One tbsp. of honey

Method:

1. Add almonds, dragon fruit, coconut, and chocolate chips in a high power blender. Blend until smooth.

2. Add yogurt, pineapple, and honey. Blend well.

3. Serve with chunks of dragon fruit from the top.

Kefir Blueberry Smoothie

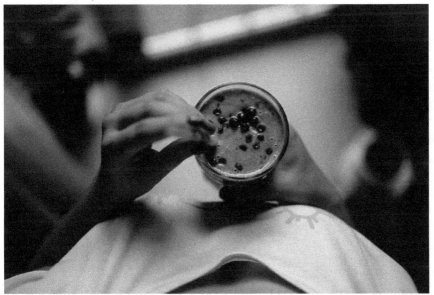

Total Prep & Cooking Time: Fifteen minutes

Yields: Two servings

Nutrition Facts: Calories: 304.2 | Protein: 7.3g | Carbs: 41.3g | Fat: 13.2g | Fiber: 4.6g

Ingredients

- Half cup of kefir
- One cup of blueberries (frozen)
- Half banana (cubed)
- One tbsp. of almond butter
- Two tsps. of honey

Method:

1. Add blueberries, banana cubes, and kefir in a blender.

2. Blend until smooth.

3. Add honey and almond butter.

4. Pulse the smoothie for a few times.

5. Serve immediately.

Ginger Fruit Smoothie

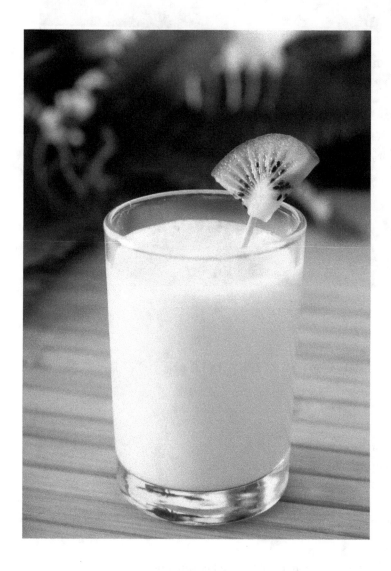

Total Prep & Cooking Time: Fifteen minutes

Yields: Two servings

Nutrition Facts: Calories: 160.2 | Protein: 1.9g | Carbs: 41.3g | Fat: 0.7g | Fiber: 5.6g

Ingredients

- One-fourth cup of each
  - Blueberries (frozen)
  - Green grapes (seedless)
- Half cup of green apple (chopped)
- One cup of water
- Three strawberries
- One piece of ginger
- One tbsp. of agave nectar

Method:

1. Add blueberries, grapes, and water in a blender. Blend the ingredients.

2. Add green apple, strawberries, agave nectar, and ginger. Blend for making thick slushy.

3. Serve immediately.

Fruit Batido

Total Prep & Cooking Time: Fifteen minutes

Yields: Six servings

Nutrition Facts: Calories: 129.3 | Protein: 4.2g | Carbs: 17.6g | Fat: 4.6g | Fiber: 0.6g

Ingredients

- One can of evaporated milk
- One cup of papaya (chopped)
- One-fourth cup of white sugar
- One tsp. of vanilla extract
- One tsp. of cinnamon (ground)
- One tray of ice cubes

Method:

1. Add papaya, white sugar, cinnamon, and vanilla extract in a food processor. Blend the ingredients until smooth.

2. Add milk and ice cubes. Blend for making slushy.

3. Serve immediately.

Banana Peanut Butter Smoothie
Total Prep & Cooking Time: Ten minutes

Yields: Four servings

Nutrition Facts: Calories: 332 | Protein: 13.2g | Carbs: 35.3g | Fat: 17.8g | Fiber: 3.9g

Ingredients

- Two bananas (cubed)
- Two cups of milk
- Half cup of peanut butter
- Two tbsps. of honey
- Two cups of ice cubes

Method:

1. Add banana cubes and peanut butter in a blender. Blend for making a smooth paste.

2. Add milk, ice cubes, and honey. Blend the ingredients until smooth.

3. Serve with banana chunks from the top.

Chapter 2: Breakfast Smoothies

Smoothie forms an essential part of breakfast in the smoothie diet plan. Here are some breakfast smoothie recipes for you that can be included in your daily breakfast plan.

Berry Banana Smoothie

Total Prep & Cooking Time: Twenty minutes

Yields: Two servings

Nutrition Facts: Calories: 330 | Protein: 6.7g | Carbs: 56.3g | Fat: 13.2g | Fiber: 5.5g

Ingredients

- One cup of each
  - Strawberries
  - Peaches (cubed)
  - Apples (cubed)
- One banana (cubed)
- Two cups of vanilla ice cream
- Half cup of ice cubes
- One-third cup of milk

Method:

1. Place strawberries, peaches, banana, and apples in a blender. Pulse the ingredients.

2. Add milk, ice cream, and ice cubes. Blend the smoothie until frothy and smooth.

3. Serve with a scoop of ice cream from the top.

Berry Surprise

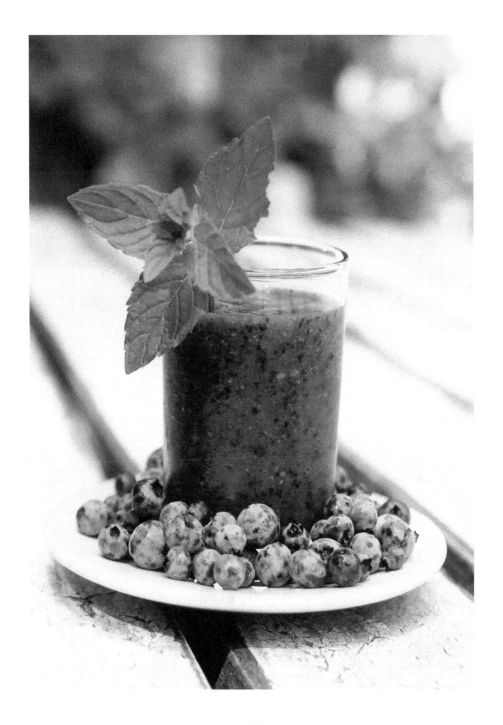

Total Prep & Cooking Time: Ten minutes

Yields: Two servings

Nutrition Facts: Calories: 164.2 | Protein: 1.2g | Carbs: 40.2g | Fat: 0.4g | Fiber: 4.8g

Ingredients

- One cup of strawberries
- Half cup of pineapple cubes
- One-third cup of raspberries
- Two tbsps. of limeade concentrate (frozen)

Method:

1. Combine pineapple cubes, strawberries, and raspberries in a food processor. Blend the ingredients until smooth.

2. Add the frozen limeade and blend again.

3. Divide the smoothie in glasses and serve immediately.

Coconut Matcha Smoothie

Total Prep & Cooking Time: Twenty minutes

Yields: Two servings

Nutrition Facts: Calories: 362 | Protein: 7.2g | Carbs: 70.1g | Fat: 8.7g | Fiber: 12.1g

Ingredients

- One large banana
- One cup of frozen mango cubes
- Two leaves of kale (torn)
- Three tbsps. of white beans (drained)
- Two tbsps. of shredded coconut (unsweetened)
- Half tsp. of matcha green tea (powder)
- Half cup of water

Method:

1. Add cubes of mango, banana, white beans, and kale in a blender. Blend all the ingredients until frothy and smooth.

2. Add shredded coconut, white beans, water, and green tea powder. Blend for thirty seconds.

3. Serve with shredded coconut from the top.

Cantaloupe Frenzy

Total Prep & Cooking Time: Ten minutes

Yields: Three servings

Nutrition Facts: Calories: 108.3 | Protein: 1.6g | Carbs: 26.2g | Fat: 0.2g | Fiber: 1.6g

Ingredients

- One cantaloupe (seeded, chopped)
- Three tbsps. of white sugar
- Two cups of ice cubes

Method:

1. Place the chopped cantaloupe along with white sugar in a blender. Puree the mixture.

2. Add cubes of ice and blend again.

3. Pour the smoothie in serving glasses. Serve immediately.

Berry Lemon Smoothie

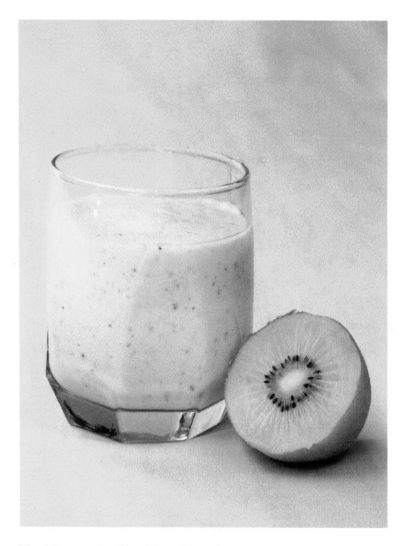

Total Prep & Cooking Time: Ten minutes

Yields: Four servings

Nutrition Facts: Calories: 97.2 | Protein: 5.4g | Carbs: 19.4g | Fat: 0.4g | Fiber: 1.8g

Ingredients

- Eight ounces of blueberry yogurt
- One and a half cup of milk (skim)
- One cup of ice cubes
- Half cup of blueberries
- One-third cup of strawberries
- One tsp. of lemonade mix

Method:

1. Add blueberry yogurt, skim milk, blueberries, and strawberries in a food processor. Blend the ingredients until smooth.

2. Add lemonade mix and ice cubes. Pulse the mixture for making a creamy and smooth smoothie.

3. Divide the smoothie in glasses and serve.

Orange Glorious

Total Prep & Cooking Time: Ten minutes

Yields: Four servings

Nutrition Facts: Calories: 212 | Protein: 3.4g | Carbs: 47.3g | Fat: 1.5g | Fiber: 0.5g

Ingredients

- Six ounces of orange juice concentrate (frozen)
- One cup of each
  - Water
  - Milk
- Half cup of white sugar
- Twelve ice cubes
- One tsp. of vanilla extract

Method:

1. Combine orange juice concentrate, white sugar, milk, and water in a blender.

2. Add vanilla extract and ice cubes. Blend the mixture until smooth.

3. Pour the smoothie in glasses and enjoy!

Grapefruit Smoothie

Total Prep & Cooking Time: Ten minutes

Yields: Two servings

Nutrition Facts: Calories: 200.3 | Protein: 4.7g | Carbs: 46.3g | Fat: 1.2g | Fiber: 7.6g

Ingredients

- Three grapefruits (peeled)
- One cup of water
- Three ounces of spinach
- Six ice cubes
- Half-inch piece of ginger
- One tsp. of flax seeds

Method:

1. Combine spinach, grapefruit, and ginger in a high power blender. Blend until smooth.

2. Add water, flax seeds, and ice cubes. Blend smooth.

3. Pour the smoothie in glasses and serve.

Sour Smoothie

Total Prep & Cooking Time: Ten minutes

Yields: Two servings

Nutrition Facts: Calories: 102.6 | Protein: 2.3g | Carbs: 30.2g | Fat: 0.7g | Fiber: 7.9g

Ingredients

- One cup of ice cubes
- Two fruit limes (peeled)
- One orange (peeled)
- One lemon (peeled)
- One kiwi (peeled)
- One tsp. of honey

Method:

1. Add fruit limes, lemon, orange, and kiwi in a food processor. Blend until frothy and smooth.

2. Add cubes of ice and honey. Pulse the ingredients.

3. Divide the smoothie in glasses and enjoy!

Ginger Orange Smoothie

Total Prep & Cooking Time: Ten minutes

Yields: One serving

Nutrition Facts: Calories: 115.6 | Protein: 2.2g | Carbs: 27.6g | Fat: 1.3g | Fiber: 5.7g

Ingredients

- One large orange
- Two carrots (peeled, cut in chunks)
- Half cup of each
  - Red grapes
  - Ice cubes
- One-fourth cup of water
- One-inch piece of ginger

Method:

1. Combine carrots, grapes, and orange in a high power blender. Blend until frothy and smooth.

2. Add ice cubes, ginger, and water. Blend the ingredients for thirty seconds.

3. Serve immediately.

Cranberry Smoothie

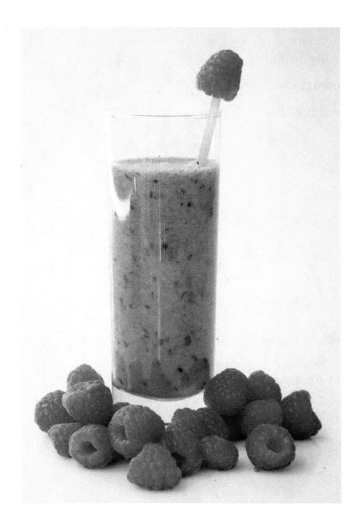

Total Prep & Cooking Time: One hour and ten minutes

Yields: Two servings

Nutrition Facts: Calories: 155.9 | Protein: 2.2g | Carbs: 33.8g | Fat: 1.6g | Fiber: 5.2g

Ingredients

- One cup of almond milk
- Half cup of mixed berries (frozen)
- One-third cup of cranberries
- One banana

Method:

1. Blend mixed berries, banana, and cranberries in a high power food processor. Blend until smooth.

2. Add almond milk and blend again for twenty seconds.

3. Refrigerate the prepared smoothie for one hour.

4. Serve chilled.

Creamsicle Smoothie

Total Prep & Cooking Time: Ten minutes

Yields: Two servings

Nutrition Facts: Calories: 121.3 | Protein: 4.7g | Carbs: 19.8g | Fat: 2.5g | Fiber: 0.3g

Ingredients

- One cup of orange juice
- One and a half cup of crushed ice
- Half cup of milk
- One tsp. of white sugar

Method:

1. Blend milk, orange juice, white sugar, and ice in a high power blender.

2. Keep blending until there is no large chunk of ice. Try to keep the consistency of slushy.

3. Serve immediately.

Sunshine Smoothie

Total Prep & Cooking Time: Thirty minutes

Yields: Four servings

Nutrition Facts: Calories: 176.8 | Protein: 4.2g | Carbs: 39.9g | Fat: 1.3g | Fiber: 3.9g

Ingredients

- Two nectarines (pitted, quartered)
- One banana (cut in chunks)
- One orange (peeled, quartered)
- One cup of vanilla yogurt
- One-third cup of orange juice
- One tbsp. of honey

Method:

1. Add banana chunks, nectarines, and orange in a blender. Blender for two minutes.

2. Add vanilla yogurt, honey, and orange juice. Blend the ingredients until frothy and smooth.

3. Pour the smoothie in glasses and serve.

Chapter 3: Vegetable Smoothies

Apart from fruit smoothies, vegetable smoothies can also provide you with essential nutrients. In fact, vegetable smoothies are tasty as well. So, here are some vegetable smoothie recipes for you.

Mango Kale Berry Smoothie
Total Prep & Cooking Time: Ten minutes

Yields: Four servings

Nutrition Facts: Calories: 117.3 | Protein: 3.1g | Carbs: 22.6g | Fat: 3.6g | Fiber: 6.2g

Ingredients

- One cup of orange juice
- One-third cup of kale
- One and a half cup of mixed berries (frozen)
- Half cup of mango chunks
- One-fourth cup of water
- Two tbsps. of chia seeds

Method:

1. Take a high power blender and add kale, orange juice, berries, mango chunks, chia seeds, and half a cup of water.

2. Blend the ingredients on high settings until smooth.

3. In case the smoothie is very thick, you can adjust the consistency by adding more water.

4. Pour the smoothie in glasses and serve.

Breakfast Pink Smoothie

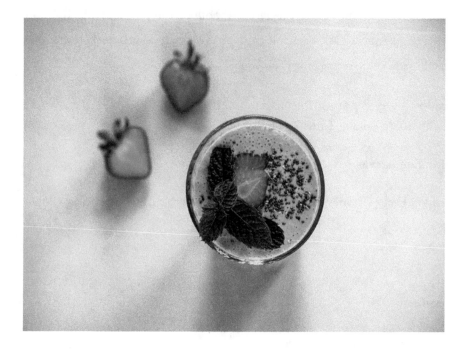

Total Prep & Cooking Time: Ten minutes

Yields: Two servings

Nutrition Facts: Calories: 198.3 | Protein: 12.3g | Carbs: 6.3g | Fat: 4.5g | Fiber: 8.8g

Ingredients

- One and a half cup of strawberries (frozen)
- One cup of raspberries
- One orange (peeled)

- Two carrots
- Two cups of coconut milk (light)
- One small beet (quartered)

Method:

1. Add strawberries, raspberries, and orange in a blender. Blend until frothy and smooth.

2. Add beet, carrots, and coconut milk.

3. Blend again for one minute.

4. Divide the smoothie in glasses and serve.

Butternut Squash Smoothie

Total Prep & Cooking Time: Five minutes

Yields: Four servings

Nutrition Facts: Calories: 127.3 | Protein: 2.3g | Carbs: 32.1g | Fat: 1.2g | Fiber: 0.6g

Ingredients

- Two cups of almond milk
- One-fourth cup of nut butter (of your choice)
- One cup of water
- One and a half cup of butternut squash (frozen)
- Two ripe bananas
- One tsp. of cinnamon (ground)
- Two tbsps. of hemp protein
- Half cup of strawberries
- One tbsp. of chia seeds
- Half tbsp. of bee pollen

Method:

1. Add butternut squash, bananas, strawberries, and almond milk in a blender. Blend until frothy and smooth.

2. Add water, nut butter, cinnamon, hemp protein, chia seeds, and bee pollen. Blend the ingredients f0r two minutes.

3. Divide the smoothie in glasses and enjoy!

Zucchini and Wild Blueberry Smoothie

Total Prep & Cooking Time: Ten minutes

Yields: Three servings

Nutrition Facts: Calories: 190.2 | Protein: 7.3g | Carbs: 27.6g | Fat: 8.1g | Fiber: 5.7g

Ingredients

- One banana
- One cup of wild blueberries (frozen)
- One-fourth cup of peas (frozen)
- Half cup of zucchini (frozen, chopped)
- One tbsp. of each
  - Hemp hearts
  - Chia seeds
  - Bee pollen
- One-third cup of almond milk
- Two tbsps. of nut butter (of your choice)
- Ten cubes of ice

Method:

1. Add blueberries, banana, peas, and zucchini in a high power blender. Blend the ingredients for two minutes.

2. Add chia seeds, hemp hearts, almond milk, bee pollen, nut butter, and ice. Blend the mixture for making a thick and smooth smoothie.

3. Pour the smoothie in glasses and serve with chopped blueberries from the top.

Cauliflower and Blueberry Smoothie

Total Prep & Cooking Time: Five minutes

Yields: Two servings

Nutrition Facts: Calories: 201.9 | Protein: 7.1g | Carbs: 32.9g | Fat: 10.3g | Fiber: 4.6g

Ingredients

- One Clementine (peeled)
- Three-fourth cup of cauliflower (frozen)
- Half cup of wild blueberries (frozen)
- One cup of Greek yogurt
- One tbsp. of peanut butter
- Bunch of spinach

Method:

1. Add cauliflower, Clementine, and blueberries in a blender. Blend for one minute.

2. Add peanut butter, spinach, and yogurt. Pulse the ingredients for two minutes until smooth.

3. Divide the prepared smoothie in glasses and enjoy!

Immunity Booster Smoothie

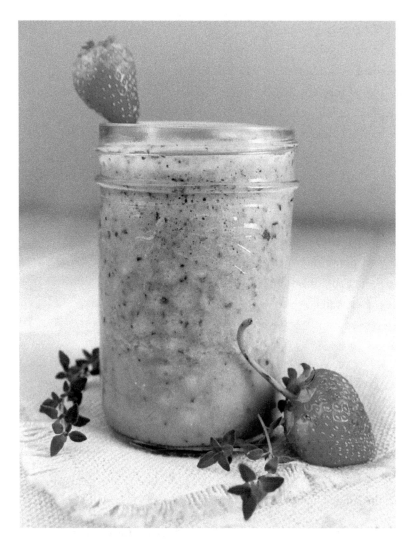

Total Prep & Cooking Time: Ten minutes

Yields: Two servings

Nutrition Facts: Calories: 301.9 | Protein: 5.4g | Carbs: 70.7g | Fat: 4.3g | Fiber: 8.9g

Ingredients

For the orange layer:

- One persimmon (quartered)
- One ripe mango (chopped)
- One lime (juiced)
- One tbsp. of nut butter (of your choice)
- Half tsp. of turmeric powder
- One pinch of cayenne pepper
- One cup of coconut milk

For the pink layer:

- One small beet (cubed)
- One cup of berries (frozen)
- One pink grapefruit (quartered)
- One-fourth cup of pomegranate juice
- Half cup of water
- Six leaves of mint
- One tsp. of honey

Method:

1. Add the ingredients for the orange layer in a blender. Blend for making a smooth liquid.

2. Pour the orange liquid evenly in serving glasses.

3. Add the pink layer ingredients in a blender. Blend for making a smooth liquid.

4. Pour the pink liquid slowly over the orange layer.

5. Pour in such a way so that both layers can be differentiated.

6. Serve immediately.

Ginger, Carrot, and Turmeric Smoothie

Total Prep & Cooking Time: Forty minutes

Yields: Two servings

Nutrition Facts: Calories: 140 | Protein: 2.6g | Carbs: 30.2g | Fat: 2.2g | Fiber: 5.6g

Ingredients

For carrot juice:

- Two cups of water
- Two and a half cups of carrots

For smoothie:

- One ripe banana (sliced)
- One cup of pineapple (frozen, cubed)
- Half tbsp. of ginger
- One-fourth tsp. of turmeric (ground)
- Half cup of carrot juice
- One tbsp. of lemon juice
- One-third cup of almond milk

Method:

1.   Add water and carrots in a high power blender. Blend on high settings for making smooth juice.

2.   Take a dish towel and strain the juice over a bowl. Squeeze the towel for taking out most of the juice.

3.   Add the ingredients for the smoothie in a blender and blend until frothy and creamy.

4.   Add carrot juice and blend again.

5.   Pour the smoothie in glasses and serve.

Romaine Mango Smoothie

Total Prep & Cooking Time: Five minutes

Yields: Two servings

Nutrition Facts: Calories: 117.3 | Protein: 2.6g | Carbs: 30.2g | Fat: 0.9g | Fiber: 4.2g

Ingredients

- Sixteen ounces of coconut water
- Two mangoes (pitted)
- One head of romaine (chopped)
- One banana
- One orange (peeled)
- Two cups of ice

Method:

1. Add mango, romaine, orange, and banana in a high power blender. Blend the ingredients until frothy and smooth.

2. Add coconut water and ice cubes. Blend for one minute.

3. Pour the prepared smoothie in glasses and serve.

Fig Zucchini Smoothie

Total Prep & Cooking Time: Ten minutes

Yields: Two servings

Nutrition Facts: Calories: 243.3 | Protein: 14.4g | Carbs: 74.3g | Fat: 27.6g | Fiber: 9.3g

Ingredients

- Half cup of cashew nuts
- One tsp. of cinnamon (ground)
- Two figs (halved)
- One banana
- Half tsp. of ginger (minced)
- One-third tsp. of honey
- One-fourth cup of ice cubes
- One pinch of salt
- Two tsps. of vanilla extract
- Three-fourth cup of water
- One cup of zucchini (chopped)

Method:

1. Add all the listed ingredients in a high power blender. Blend for two minutes until creamy and smooth.

2. Pour the smoothie in serving glasses and serve.

Carrot Peach Smoothie

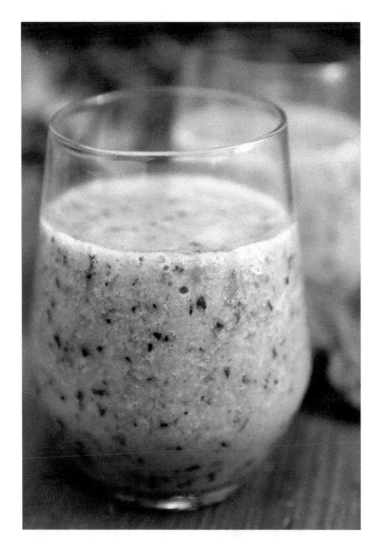

Total Prep & Cooking Time: Ten minutes

Yields: Two servings

Nutrition Facts: Calories: 191.2 | Protein: 11.2g | Carbs: 34.6g | Fat: 2.7g | Fiber: 5.4g

Ingredients

- Two cups of peach
- One cup of baby carrots
- One banana (frozen)
- Two tbsps. of Greek yogurt
- One and a half cup of coconut water
- One tbsp. of honey

Method:

1. Add peach, baby carrots, and banana in a high power blender. Blend on high settings for one minute.

2. Add Greek yogurt, honey, and coconut water. Give the mixture a whizz.

3. Pour the smoothie in glasses and serve.

Sweet Potato and Mango Smoothie

Total Prep & Cooking Time: Ten minutes

Yields: Two servings

Nutrition Facts: Calories: 133.3 | Protein: 3.6g | Carbs: 28.6g | Fat: 1.3g | Fiber: 6.2g

Ingredients

- One small sweet potato (cooked, smashed)
- Half cup of mango chunks (frozen)
- Two cups of coconut milk
- One tbsp. of chia seeds
- Two tsps. of maple syrup
- A handful of ice cubes

Method:

1. Add mango chunks and sweet potato in a high power blender. Blend until frothy and smooth.

2. Add chia seeds, coconut milk, ice cubes, and maple syrup. Blend again for one minute.

3. Divide the smoothie in glasses and serve.

Carrot Cake Smoothie

Total Prep & Cooking Time: Ten minutes

Yields: Two servings

Nutrition Facts: Calories: 289.3 | Protein: 3.6g | Carbs: 47.8g | Fat: 1.3g | Fiber: 0.6g

Ingredients

- One cup of carrots (chopped)
- One banana
- Half cup of almond milk
- One cup of Greek yogurt
- One tbsp. of maple syrup
- One tsp. of cinnamon (ground)
- One-fourth tsp. of nutmeg
- Half tsp. of ginger (ground)
- A handful of ice cubes

Method

1. Add banana, carrots, and almond milk in a blender. Blend until frothy and smooth.

2. Add yogurt, cinnamon, maple syrup, ginger, nutmeg, and ice cubes. Blend again for two minutes.

3. Divide the smoothie in serving glasses and serve.

Notes:

- You can add more ice cubes and turn the smoothie into slushy.

- You can store the leftover smoothie in the freezer for two days.

Chapter 4: Green Smoothies

Green smoothies can help in the process of detoxification as well as weight loss. Here are some easy-to-make green smoothie recipes for you.

Kale Avocado Smoothie

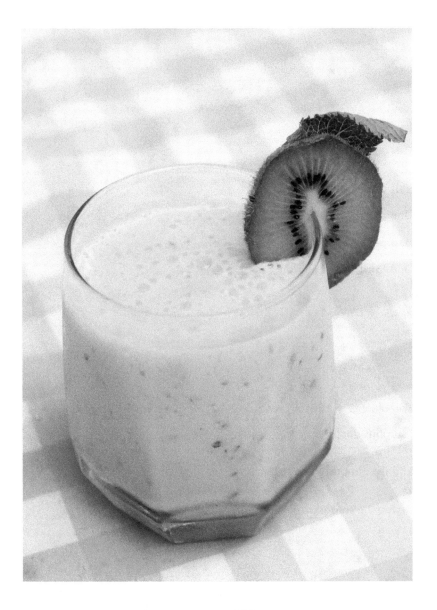

Total Prep & Cooking Time: Ten minutes

Yields: Two servings

Nutrition Facts: Calories: 401 | Protein: 11.2g | Carbs: 64.6g | Fat: 17.3g | Fiber: 10.2g

Ingredients

- One banana (cut in chunks)
- Half cup of blueberry yogurt
- One cup of kale (chopped)
- Half ripe avocado
- One-third cup of almond milk

Method:

1. Add blueberry, banana, avocado, and kale in a blender. Blend for making a smooth mixture.

2. Add the almond milk and blend again.

3. Divide the smoothie in glasses and serve.

Celery Pineapple Smoothie

Total Prep & Cooking Time: Ten minutes

Yields: Two servings

Nutrition Facts: Calories: 112 | Protein: 2.3g | Carbs: 3.6g | Fat: 1.2g | Fiber: 3.9g

Ingredients

- Three celery stalks (chopped)
- One cup of cubed pineapple
- One banana
- One pear
- Half cup of almond milk
- One tsp. of honey

Method:

1. Add celery stalks, pear, banana, and cubes of pineapple in a food processor. Blend until frothy and smooth.

2. Add honey and almond milk. Blend for two minutes.

3. Pour the smoothie in serving glasses and enjoy!

Cucumber Mango and Lime Smoothie

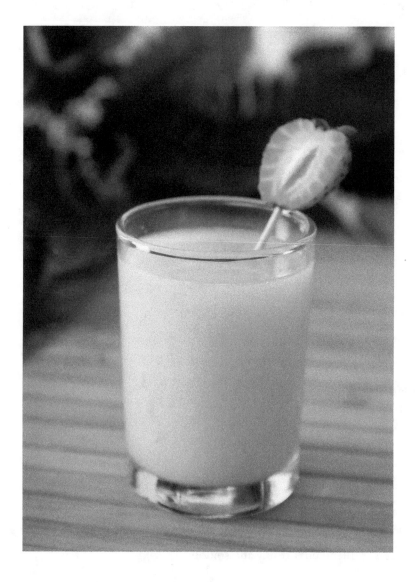

Total Prep & Cooking Time: Ten minutes

Yields: Two servings

Nutrition Facts: Calories: 165 | Protein: 2.2g | Carbs: 32.5g | Fat: 4.2g | Fiber: 3.7g

Ingredients

- One cup of ripe mango (frozen, cubed)
- Six cubes of ice
- Half cup of baby spinach leaves
- Two leaves of mint
- Two tsps. of lime juice
- Half cucumber (chopped)
- Three-fourth cup of coconut milk
- One-eighth tsp. of cayenne pepper

Method:

1. Add mango cubes, spinach leaves, and cucumber in a high power blender. Blend until frothy and smooth.

2. Add mint leaves, lime juice, coconut milk, cayenne pepper, and ice cubes. Process the ingredients until smooth.

3. Pour the smoothie in glasses and serve.

Kale, Melon, and Broccoli Smoothie

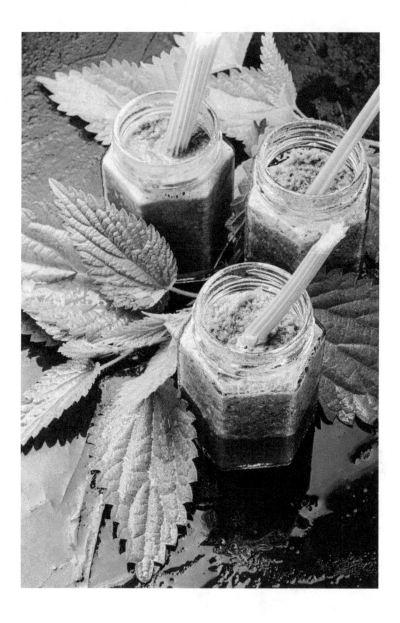

Total Prep & Cooking Time: Ten minutes

Yields: One serving

Nutrition Facts: Calories: 96.3 | Protein: 2.3g | Carbs: 24.3g | Fat: 1.2g | Fiber: 2.6g

Ingredients

- Eight ounces of honeydew melon
- One handful of kale
- Two ounces of broccoli florets
- One cup of coconut water
- Two sprigs of mint
- Two dates
- Half cup of lime juice
- Eight cubes of ice

Method:

1. Add kale, melon, and broccoli in a food processor. Whizz the ingredients for blending.

2. Add mint leaves and coconut water. Blend again.

3. Add lime juice, dates, and ice cubes. Blend the ingredients until smooth and creamy.

4. Pour the smoothie in a smoothie glass. Enjoy!

Kiwi Spinach Smoothie

Total Prep & Cooking Time: Ten minutes

Yields: Two servings

Nutrition Facts: Calories: 102 | Protein: 3.6g | Carbs: 21.3g | Fat: 2.2g | Fiber: 3.1g

Ingredients

- One kiwi (cut in chunks)
- One banana (cut in chunks)
- One cup of spinach leaves
- Three-fourth cup of almond milk
- One tbsp. of chia seeds
- Four cubes of ice

Method:

1. Add banana, kiwi, and spinach leaves in a blender. Blend the ingredients until smooth.

2. Add chia seeds, ice cubes, and almond milk. Blend again for one minute.

3. Pour the smoothie in serving glasses and serve.

Avocado Smoothie

Total Prep & Cooking Time: Ten minutes

Yields: Two servings

Nutrition Facts: Calories: 345 | Protein: 9.1g | Carbs: 47.8g | Fat: 16.9g | Fiber: 6.7g

Ingredients

- One ripe avocado (halved, pitted)
- One cup of milk
- Half cup of vanilla yogurt
- Eight cubes of ice
- Three tbsps. of honey

Method:

1. Add avocado, vanilla yogurt, and milk in a blender. Blend the ingredients until frothy and smooth.

2. Add honey and ice cubes. Blend the ingredients for making a smooth mixture.

3. Serve immediately.

CPSIA information can be obtained
at www.ICGtesting.com
Printed in the USA
LVHW081812161020
669013LV00003B/39